Feline Practice

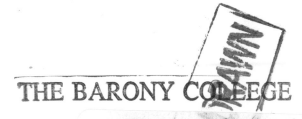

The *In Practice* Handbooks Series

Series Editor: Edward Boden

Past and present members of *In Practice* Editorial Board

Titles in print:
Feline Practice
Canine Practice
Equine Practice

Forthcoming titles:
Bovine Practice
Sheep and Goat Practice
Swine Practice

The *In Practice* Handbooks

Feline Practice

Edited by E. Boden
Executive Editor, *In Practice*

Baillière Tindall

LONDON   PHILADELPHIA   TORONTO   SYDNEY   TOKYO

Baillière Tindall   24–28 Oval Road
W.B. Saunders   London NW1 7DX

The Curtis Center
Independence Square West
Philadelphia, PA 19106–3399, USA

55 Horner Avenue
Toronto, Ontario M8Z 4X6, Canada

Harcourt Brace Jovanovich Group
(Australia) Pty Ltd
30–52 Smidmore Street
Marrickville
NSW 2204, Australia

Harcourt Brace Jovanovich Japan Inc
Ichibancho Central Building,
22–1 Ichibancho
Chiyoda-ku, Tokyo 102, Japan

Typeset by Photo·graphics, Honiton, Devon
Printed and bound in Hong Kong by Dah Hua Printing Press Co., Ltd.

A catalogue record for this book is available from the British Library

ISBN 0–7020–1523–7

Contents

Contributors

P.G.C. Bedford, Reader in Veterinary Ophthalmology, Department of Veterinary Surgery and Obstetrics, Royal Veterinary College, University of London, London, UK

A. Blaxter, Department of Veterinary Medicine, University of Bristol, Bristol, UK

I. Burger, Waltham Centre for Pet Nutrition, Melton Mowbray, Leicestershire, UK

A.T.B. Edney, Crocket Cottage, Oakham, Leicestershire, UK

R. Evans, Department of Veterinary Medicine, University of Bristol, Bristol, UK

C. Gaskell, Department of Veterinary Pathology and Clinical Science, University of Liverpool, Liverpool, UK

R. Gaskell, Department of Veterinary Pathology and Clinical Science, University of Liverpool, Liverpool, UK

T.J. Gruffydd-Jones, Department of Veterinary Medicine, University of Bristol, Bristol, UK

D. Horrocks, Waltham Centre for Pet Nutrition, Melton Mowbray, Leicestershire, UK

O. Jarrett, Professor, Department of Veterinary Pathology, University of Glasgow Veterinary School, Glasgow, UK

J. Knowles, 45 Baalhec Road, Highbury, London, UK

K.L. Thoday, Department of Clinical Veterinary Studies, University of Edinburgh, Edinburgh, UK

Foreword

In Practice was started in 1979 as a clinical supplement to *The Veterinary Record*. Its carefully chosen, highly illustrated articles specially commissioned from leaders in their field were aimed specifically at the practitioner. They have proved extremely popular with experienced veterinarians and students alike. The editorial board, chaired for the first 10 years by Professor James Armour, was particularly concerned to emphasize differential diagnosis.

In response to consistent demand, articles from *In Practice*, updated and revised by the authors, are now published in convenient handbook form. Each book deals with a particular species or group of related animals.

E. Boden

CHAPTER 1

Feline Leukaemia Virus

OSWALD JARRETT

INTRODUCTION

The awareness of feline leukaemia virus (FeLV) as a cause of serious disease in cats has increased with the recognition that FeLV is involved in the pathogenesis of many diseases other than lymphosarcoma from which the virus was first isolated. Epidemiological studies have defined the populations of cats which are at risk from the effects of the virus and have suggested measures for the control of FeLV infections.

FeLV-RELATED DISEASES

FeLV causes lymphosarcoma and leukaemia of various types, anaemia and general immunodeficiency, and is also intimately associated with, and may well be the cause of, infertility due to early fetal death and other reproductive problems. Further associations exist between FeLV infection and both feline infectious peritonitis and feline infectious anaemia caused by *Haemobartonella felis*. However, each of these diseases may occur in the absence of FeLV infection so that the role of FeLV in their pathogenesis is not established but may be due to immunodeficiency. Table 1.1 lists the conditions associated with FeLV. If one or more of these occur in a household of cats, FeLV infection should be suspected. Jarrett (1985) has reviewed the clinico-pathological aspects of many FeLV related diseases.

Lymphosarcoma is the most common malignant tumour of cats. Table 1.2 shows the prevalence of the different types of lymphosarcoma encountered in our hospital. Different distributions have been noted elsewhere possibly because of the use of different diagnostic methods or perhaps because of the occurrence of distinct strains of FeLV in different places. Table 1.2 also indicates the important point that FeLV cannot be isolated from all cats with spontaneous lymphosarcoma; for example, the virus is present in only about one third of cases of alimentary lymphosarcoma. The relationship, if any, of FeLV to virus-negative cases of lymphosarcoma is still unproven. However, the majority of cases of lymphosarcoma which are diagnosed in FeLV-infected multiple cat households occur in cats from which FeLV may be isolated.

Table 1.1 Diseases associated with FeLV infection.

Haemopoietic tumours	
Lymphoid:	thymic lymphosarcoma
	multicentric lymphosarcoma
	alimentary lymphosarcoma
	lymphatic leukaemia
Myeloid	
Erythroid	
Anaemia	
Haemolytic	
Aplastic	
Reproductive problems	
Infertility (early fetal death)	
Abortion	
Immunodeficiency	
Pneumonia, septicaemia, gingivitis	
Haemobartonella infection	

FeLV REPLICATION

FeLV belongs to the retrovirus group which has a unique replication cycle in which a copy of the viral gene is integrated into the chromosomes of infected cells to become a "provirus". Subsequent expression of the provirus leads to the assembly of new viral particles at the cell surface by the budding process illustrated in Fig. 1.1. In this way the cell is not killed but may continue to produce virus over long periods.

The viral life cycle underlines three very important features of the pathogenesis of FeLV-related diseases. First, it is the basis of the lifelong infections which often become established following FeLV infection. Secondly, since retroviruses require cellular DNA synthesis for replication, FeLV multiplies in tissues where there are divided cells, notably in the bone marrow and in many epithelial cells throughout the body. Thirdly, it indicates that the elimination of FeLV infection from cats requires the deletion of virus-infected cells and not only clearance of free extra-cellular virus.

TRANSMISSION OF FeLV

The major source of FeLV is the chronically infected cat which may be clinically ill with a FeLV-related disease, in the incubation period of disease, or a healthy virus carrier. The virus is transmitted congenitally or by contact. In congenital infections the virus is transmitted before birth although the stage of pregnancy at which the virus infects the fetus is not known. In many cases infection of the very young embryo is

Table 1.2 The prevalence of lymphosarcoma types in cats.

Lymphosarcoma type	Frequency (%)	FeLV-positive (%)
Thymic lymphosarcoma	20	37
Multicentric lymphosarcoma	24	53
Alimentary lymphosarcoma	50	90
Lymphatic leukaemia	5	66

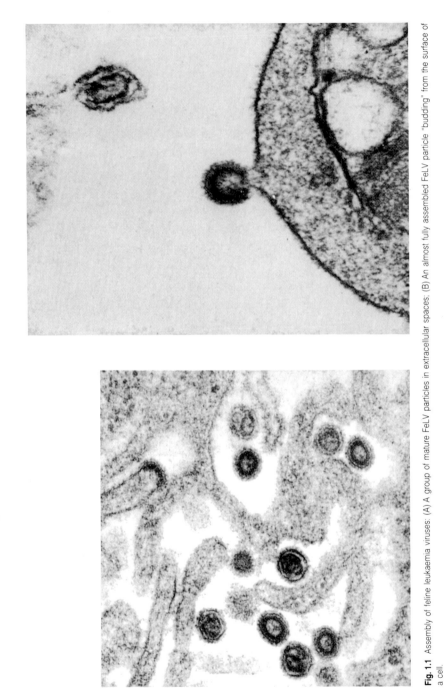

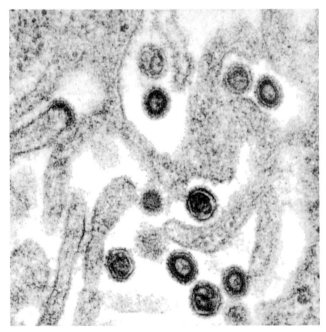

Fig. 1.1 Assembly of feline leukaemia viruses: (A) A group of mature FeLV particles in extracellular spaces; (B) An almost fully assembled FeLV particle "budding" from the surface of a cell.

likely since early fetal death is a frequent feature in infected queens. Transmission by contact occurs through virus-containing saliva and close contact is required for virus spread.

Following exposure to FeLV there appears to be two alternative longterm consequences: immunity or persistent infection. FeLV-related diseases occur in cats which have persistent infections. The incubation period from virus exposure to the appearance of clinical disease may be very long, especially in the case of lymphosarcoma, ranging from months to several years. Epidemiological studies suggest that the median incubation period for lymphosarcoma is about 3–4 years. During this time the cat appears clinically normal although it is excreting virus.

The outcome of FeLV infection is influencd by two main factors: the age at which the cat is infected and the dose of virus to which the cat is exposed. The proportion of cats which develop persistent viraemia varies according to the age at which the cat is infected. Infection early in life, either *in utero* or in the neonatal period, always results in a persistent viral infection without a detectable immune response. These cats have a very high risk of developing disease. From 4 months of age onwards the majority of cats become immune following natural FeLV infection. Another important determinant of susceptibility is the way in which cats are housed. Free-range cats infrequently become persistently infected with FeLV while large numbers of cats kept in closed communities in which the virus is enzootic develop chronic FeLV infections. The basis of this difference is probably the dose of virus. The high dose in closed communities tends to lead to persistent infections while the low dose to which free-range cats are exposed tends to immunize.

OUTCOME OF FeLV INFECTION

About 10 days after intranasal instillation of FeLV, virus is found replicating in the bone marrow, for which it has a strong affinity. From there the virus spreads in the blood to many other tissues throughout the body including the salivary gland and within 10–20 days after infection is excreted from the mouth. In the blood both virus and FeLV p27 antigen are found free in the plasma and FeLV antigen is present in the cytoplasm of the circulating polymorphonuclear leucocytes and platelets: this forms the basis of the diagnostic procedures for the virus.

Cats with persistent FeLV viraemia have a poor prognosis. In one study 85% died or were destroyed within 4 years of natural infection.

Many cats which do not develop a persistent infection following exposure to FeLV show a transient viraemia which may last from 1–8 weeks and then disappear. This is usually followed by the appearance of virus neutralizing (VN) antibodies. Other transiently infected cats show no evidence of virus in the blood but still become immune.

Immunity is the major factor influencing the outcome of FeLV infections. Antibody may appear in the serum of cats following FeLV infection. VN antibody is directed against antigens on the surface of the virus and is responsible for inactivating free virus. Cats with VN antibodies are resistant to infection with FeLV.

Newborn kittens from immune queens acquire maternal VN antibodies which protect them against exposure to large doses of FeLV. This passively acquired antibody is gradually eliminated from the kittens by about 6 weeks of age after which they enter a period of 6–7 weeks when they are still very susceptible to FeLV excreted by virus carriers. Such findings reinforce the benefit of maintaining queens and their young kittens in isolation from other cats which may be carriers of FeLV, or indeed of other feline viruses.

LATENT FeLV INFECTIONS

Of the recovered cats, some appear to eliminate the virus completely. However many harbour a latent infection in which the virus is present in a dormant state in bone marrow cells, but neither virus nor viral antigen can be isolated from the blood. This latent state is maintained by VN antibodies but when the suppressive effect of this immune response is removed, either *in vivo* by treating the cats with very high doses of corticosteroids or *in vitro* by culturing bone marrow cells obtained from the cats at biopsy, the virus is reactivated and can readily be demonstrated in the blood or culture fluid, respectively.

The proportion of cats with a latent infection falls with time, suggesting that the marrow cells in which the virus is latent are gradually eliminated. However, about 10% of cats maintain latent virus for many months, and possibly for life, so that the question arises whether these cats transmit virus to susceptible in-contact animals. What evidence there is indicates that they do not transmit virus by contact but some may transfer feline leukaemia virus to their kittens in milk (Pacitti *et al.*, 1986).

The outcome of FeLV infection may now be perceived as a spectrum ranging from persistent productive infection with viraemia at one end, through focal productive infection with release of antigen but not virus into the blood, to controlled latent infection with no plasma virus or antigen, and then complete elimination of virus at the other end.

EPIDEMIOLOGY OF FeLV

Two distinct epidemiological patterns of FeLV infection have been defined: multi-cat house and single-cat house patterns, the main characteristics of which are indicated in Table 1.3.

The basis of the differences between these situations is probably the dose of virus to which the cat is exposed in

Table 1.3 Epidemiology patterns in FeLV infections.

Open house
Free range cats
High prevalence of anti-FOCMA antibodies (50%)
Low prevalence of virus neutralizing antibodies (5%)
Low prevalence of persistent viraemia (<5%)
Low incidence of FeLV-related disease

Closed house
Isolated cats
High prevalence of anti-FOCMA antibodies (80%)
High prevalence of virus neutralizing antibodies (40%)
High prevalence of persistent viraemia (40%)
High incidence of FeLV-related disease

each. In closed multi-cat households in which FeLV is enzootic, susceptible cats are often in intimate contact with excreting cats and hence the dose of virus to which they are exposed is high. By contrast, free-range cats are in frequent but brief contact with their neighbours so that the dose of virus transmitted is likely to be small.

In closed FeLV-infected multi-cat households the prevalence of antibodies is high and active FeLV viraemia is very common. When FeLV is introduced, usually in the form of an infected carrier cat, all cats which are in contact become infected within a short period of time. On average 60–70% of cats recover from the infection and most develop VN antibodies. Cats with VN antibodies are resistant to reinfection with FeLV. However, the remaining 30–40% of the cats become persistently viraemic.

In free-range urban and suburban cat populations FeLV infection is also common as determined by the prevalence of antibodies, but FeLV-related disease is uncommon (Hosie *et al.*, 1989). There is a good correlation between the extent of roaming and the proportion with antibody in that very few young kittens (5%) but many stray cats (70%) have antibody. However, the occurrence of active FeLV viraemia is rare in cats in this population with an approximate prevalence of up to 5% and consequently the incidence of lymphosarcoma is relatively low.

PUBLIC HEALTH ASPECTS

All available evidence suggests that FeLV is not transmissible to man. Cases of leukaemia have been found concurrently in pets and owners but these have not been sufficiently common to conclude that their occurrence was due to anything more than chance. Further, analysis by sensitive assay of leukaemic material from human patients has failed to detect FeLV antigen and serological or virological evidence for FeLV infection of possible high risk persons such as cat owners or veterinarians who handle, knowingly or not, cats which are excreting the virus, or laboratory personnel working with large quantities of FeLV, is similarly lacking.

DIAGNOSIS AND CONTROL OF FeLV INFECTIONS

Control of FeLV infection depends on the detection of carriers by demonstrating virus or viral antigen in the blood. Three diagnostic tests for FeLV are available: virus isolation, immunofluorescence or ELISA. Of these, the latter is available in kit form and can be performed by veterinary practitioners in their own laboratories.

Comparison of these three methods indicates that while virus isolation and immunofluorescence give essentially identical results, there is a degree of discordance between these two tests and ELISA. Thus 10% of samples which are positive by ELISA are negative by virus isolation or immunofluorescence (Jarrett *et al.*, 1982). This finding is worrying because FeLV-positive cats often face euthanasia.

Several questions arise about these "discordant" cats. First, do they become viraemic? Follow-up studies indicate that only a very small proportion become viraemic, and those that do so as the result of (re)infection with feline leukaemia virus. Most of the cats maintain the "discordant" state.

Second, would these cats develop a disease which might be related to feline leukaemia virus infection? There is no evidence that they do since most remained healthy after 3 years of observation. Third, do they transmit virus to in-contact cats? Again, there is no evidence for spread of virus from these cats to in-contact animals.

The method of control which is used is shown in Table 1.4. This involves the detection and removal of FeLV-positive cats, either by isolation, re-homing or euthanasia. An important part of the protocol is the retesting of cats after 12 weeks. The reason for retesting virus-negative cats is to ensure that they were not incubating the infection at the time of the initial sampling when the virus might not yet have been present in the blood. Whether or not to keep and retest virus-positive cats depends on the individual situation. Of the cats which initially prove positive, the vast majority will have a permanent infection. However, it is known that by chance a few will be sampled during a transient viraemia after which the cats will recover and isolation and retesting of the FeLV-positive cats may establish if this is the case or not. There is always a risk to susceptible cats of maintaining FeLV-positive and negative cats in the same household unless isolation is stringent. This should be taken into account when advising on measures of control. Important factors which influence the decision include the extent of disease in the household, the number of cats involved, the value of the cats and the housing resources which are available.

A continuing anxiety in households from which the virus has been eliminated or which are found to be FeLV-free is that FeLV might be (re)introduced. All cats which subsequently come into the house must be tested before, or immediately on, entry and ideally they should then be isolated for 12 weeks and tested again before being allowed to mix freely with existing FeLV-negative cats. Cats from closed households may come into contact with others at show and at stud. The extent of contact between cats at shows is unlikely to be sufficient for FeLV to be transmitted. Several studies suggest that the FeLV-infected stud cat is an important means of spread of FeLV and many owners of stud cats have them tested at intervals of 6–12 months and insist that visiting queens be FeLV-negative. Breeding cats may also be tested for VN antibodies to determine whether they are likely to be immune for FeLV infection.

VACCINATION

Vaccines against FeLV which are available in some countries are not yet on sale in the UK. The manufacturers claim a protection factor of 70–80% for their products but there is

Table 1.4 Control of FeLV infections in closed households.

Test all cats (or all permanent stock)
Remove or isolate viraemic cats. Isolate
     FeLV-negative cats.
Quarantine: no introductions or removals
Disinfect premises of negative cats
Retest cats after 12 weeks
Test introductions before entry
Retest breeding cats annually

controversy about the efficacy of some of these vaccines and there are no field studies which unequivocally demonstrate that vaccination is worthwhile.

REFERENCES AND FURTHER READING

Hosie, M. J., Robertson, C. & Jarrett, O. (1989). *Veterinary Record* **128**, 293.
Jarrett, O. (1985). In *Feline Medicine and Therapeutics* (eds E. A. Chandler, C. J. Gaskell & A. D. R. Hilbery), pp. 271–283. Blackwell, Oxford.
Jarrett, O., Golder, M. C. & Weijer, K. (1982). *Veterinary Record* **110**, 325.
Pacitti, A. M., Jarrett, O. & Hay, D. (1986). *Veterinary Record* **118**, 381.

CHAPTER 2

Respiratory Diseases of Cats

CHRIS GASKELL AND ROSALIND GASKELL

INTRODUCTION

Respiratory disease accounts for about 10% of feline cases seen in practice and is dominated by viral upper respiratory tract infection or "cat 'flu". Conditions involving the pleural cavity are not uncommon while diseases of the lower airway and lungs are numerically much less important.

UPPER RESPIRATORY TRACT (URT) DISEASE

"CAT 'FLU" AND CHRONIC RHINITIS

Aetiology and clinical signs

Various agents have been implicated in the aetiology of this disease but it has been estimated that about 80% of cases are caused by either feline viral rhinotracheitis (FVR) virus (feline herpesvirus 1) or feline calicivirus (FCV).

Feline viral rhinotracheitis (FVR)

FVR is generally a severe URT disease, particularly in young, susceptible animals (Fig. 2.1). After an incubation period of 2–10 days, early signs include depression, pyrexia, inappetence, paroxysmal sneezing and sometimes hypersalivation, followed rapidly by marked ocular and nasal discharges, conjunctivitis, and sometimes coughing. Ulcerative keratitis may also develop. A leucocytosis with a shift to the left is present throughout the course of the disease. Occasionally with FVR but more commonly with FCV infection, lingual ulceration may be seen. Sometimes in younger or immunosuppressed individuals the disease may generalize. Fatalities most often result from dehydration and also secondary bacterial infection which may lead to bronchopneumonia. Signs generally resolve within 2–3 weeks but in some cats the severe necrosis and ulceration of the mucous membranes, particularly in the turbinate regions seen in the acute phase of the disease, leads to permanently damaged areas of mucosa which are then prone to recurrent microbial infection. In some cases persistent or recurrent signs may follow recrudescence of viral shedding in carrier cats.

Feline calicivirus infection (FCV)

FCV infection is typically milder than FVR, although there are a large number of strains of feline calicivirus in comparison with the single strain of FVR. These can cause a spectrum of disease ranging from a severe URT syndrome similar to that seen with FVR to a subclinical infection. Mouth ulceration, however, is a frequent and characteristic feature of FCV infection (Fig. 2.2). Indeed, in many cases it may appear as the only clinical sign. Ulcers may occur on the tongue, hard palate and external nares.

General malaise is usually less marked than in FVR and ocular and nasal discharges are not as copious. Some strains of calicivirus produce a primary interstitial pneumonia and dyspnoea may be a feature, and some strains may induce a febrile "limping" syndrome, often with no accompanying URT

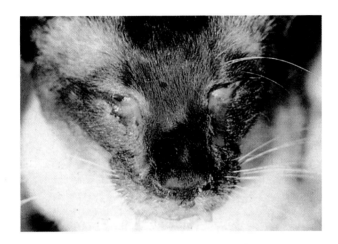

Fig. 2.1
A cat showing signs
of feline viral
rhinotracheitis (FVR).

signs. There is also an association between chronic stomatitis and gingivitis and persistent FCV infection; though the aetiological significance of this is not known.

Diagnosis

Acute viral URT infection may be identified from the presenting clinical signs and some distinction may be made on this basis between FVR and FCV infection. If a definitive diagnosis is required, an oropharyngeal swab sample should be sent in viral transport medium to an appropriate laboratory. Where persistent conjunctivitis is the predominant feature, *Chlamydia psittaci* diagnosis should be undertaken (see *In Practice* **11**(1), 23).

Bacterial culture and sensitivity testing is important in acute cases which fail to respond to an initial course of antibiotics and in cases of chronic rhinitis. The most valuable material is obtained from the nasal chambers, after the nares have been cleaned with an antiseptic solution. Chronic rhinitis classically improves, albeit temporarily, after a prolonged course of antibiotics; failure to do so might suggest other

Table 2.1 Diseases of the upper respiratory tract.

Disease	Aetiology	Significance
Acute URT disease (cat 'flu)	Feline viral rhinotracheitis virus	Approx 40% cases, tends to be more severe
	Feline calicivirus	Approx 40% cases, possible more. Usually mild
	Feline *Chlamydia psittaci*	Approx. 30% cases of persistent conjunctivitis
	Feline reovirus	Mild disease experimentally
	Feline infectious peritonitis virus	Most likely a primary enteric pathogen, but respiratory signs also suggested by some
	Bordetella	Some laboratory colonies, significance in field unknown
	Other bacteria, e.g. *Staphs, Streps, Pasteurellae,* coliforms	Mainly secondary invaders
	Mycoplasmas	Possibly primary, mainly secondary
Chronic rhinitis, sinusitis, conjunctivitis	Bacterial infection secondary to acute viral	Relatively common and tends to persist
	Recrudescent FVR	More episodic and discharges usually less purulent
Nasal mycoses	*Cryptococcus neoformans* Maduromycosis	All uncommon
Neoplasia	Carcinomata of nose and larynx Lymphosarcoma of nose and larynx Pharyngeal polyps	

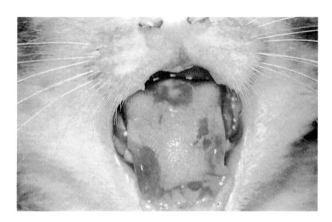

Fig. 2.2
Lingual ulceration is a characteristic feature of FCV infection. Hard palate and external nares are also sometimes affected.

much rarer diagnoses such as nasal mycoses or neoplasia. Chronically affected cats should also be screened for possible underlying feline leukaemia virus (FeLV) or feline immunodeficiency virus (FIV) infection.

Treatment

There are no antiviral drugs in widespread use at present to control FVR and FCV infection, although 5-iododeoxyuridine (IUdR) has been recommended in cases of ulcerative keratitis associated with FVR and there are other anti-herpesvirus drugs developed for use in other species which may prove useful in this disease. In general, however, recovery and the prevention of chronic sequelae may be greatly assisted by the use, initially for at least 7 days, of broad spectrum antibiotics (such as ampicillin, potentiated sulphonamide, oxytetracycline or tylosin) to control secondary bacterial infection. Since swallowing may be painful, oral dosing is best achieved with paediatric syrups. Supportive vitamin therapy (vitamins A, B, C, Abidec drops, Parke-Davis; and vitamin B_{12}) may also be helpful.

Nursing, often best done at home by the owner, is also an important factor in aiding recovery. Hospital intensive care requires scrupulous attention to hygiene to prevent cross-infection. Affected cats should be kept in a clean, warm and well-ventilated environment and kept groomed. Discharges from around the eyes and nose should be frequently wiped away and a bland ointment applied to the area to prevent excoriation. Nebulizers and steam inhalations to maintain clear airways are tolerated better by cats than the application of nasal decongestants. Corticosteroids are contraindicated because they retard the healing process and may potentiate the virus infection.

The animal should be encouraged to eat by offering strongly flavoured, aromatic foods (e.g. sardines) and in cases where oral ulceration makes eating painful, or dehydration is becoming a problem, soft liquid food should be given. Dehydration may require treatment with subcutaneous or intravenous fluids and where anorexia is prolonged, the use of a pharyngostomy tube may be indicated.

Animals should routinely be re-examined within at least a week of the start of treatment. Failure to control secondary bacterial infection may necessitate swab culture and sensitivity tests and a change of antibiotic.

Chronic rhinitis and sinusitis cases are best treated by prevention, i.e. adequate therapy in the acute phase of the disease. Once the intranasal structures are irreversibly damaged, the long term prognosis is relatively poor. Prolonged (2–3 week) antibiotic therapy, together with mucolytics (e.g. Bisolvon, Boehringer Ingelheim) may lead to only temporary remission of the clinical signs. Local infusion of antibiotics through the frontal sinuses appears to offer no advantage in the chronic phase over the oral and parenteral routes.

Radical surgical excision of diseased tissues has been used by some in cases of chronic rhinitis but radical nasal surgery is poorly tolerated by cats and the results are disappointing. Some chronically affected cats show improvement on being housed out of doors. If cats are infected with feline leukaemia or feline immunodeficiency virus then the prognosis is poor.

Epidemiology (Fig. 2.3)

The feline respiratory viruses persist in the cat population in three main ways:

FVR carrier state: Epidemiology

FCV carrier state: Epidemiology

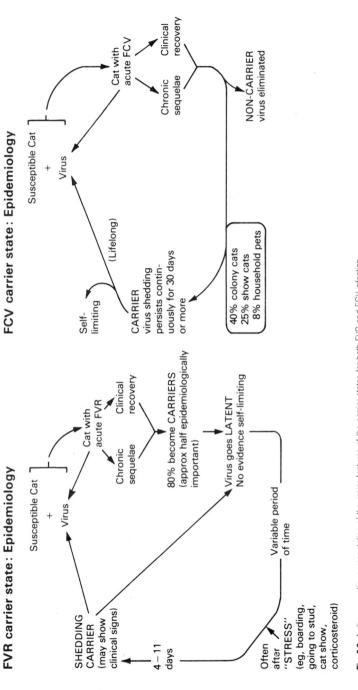

Fig. 2.3 A diagrammatic representation of the major features of the carrier states for both FVR and FCV infection.

(1) By passing directly from acutely infected to susceptible animals.

(2) By persisting in the environment for relatively short periods of time (FVR virus for up to 18 h; feline calicivirus for 8–10 days) and thus may be transmitted indirectly via infected secretions contaminating cages, feedbowls, litter trays, grooming kit and the hands, feet and clothing of personnel. Aerosol transmission is not thought to be of major significance in the transmission of the disease although it is probable that in "still air" cats can sneeze macro-droplets over a distance of about 1.5 m.

(3) By persisting in the cat itself, following recovery from the acute phase of the disease, by the establishment in certain animals of a carrier state. Such carriers are widespread in the population and are undoubtedly of importance as a source of virus, although slightly longer and more intimate contact between animals may be necessary to achieve transmission than in the acute phase of the disease.

There are no known reservoir hosts for the viruses, and vertical transmission does not normally occur.

Thus the disease mainly appears in boarding catteries, breeding colonies, stray-cat homes or other situations where a large number of cats have been brought together and infection is often introduced by the (usually) clinically normal carrier. Once endemic in a colony the disease appears mainly in the acute form in young kittens at the stage at which they lose their passive immunity. In older cats its presence may be noted by the existence of chronically affected cats suffering from persistent or recurrent rhinitis, sinusitis, conjunctivitis or bronchitis.

Control

Three types of vaccine are currently available in the UK, modified live systemic, modified live intranasal, and an inactivated systemic vaccine where the FVR component is in sub-unit form. Such vaccines are relatively successful in preventing disease, generally with few side effects in the majority of healthy, previously unexposed animals. Ideally, vaccination of the whole cat population should be the aim. Nevertheless vaccine usage should be considered in conjunction with an understanding of the epidemiology of the disease for the nature of it is such that apparent vaccine reactions and breakdowns may occur from time to time. Thus prevention and control is best approached through a combination of management and vaccination.

Individual animals should be vaccinated annually but should also be protected from contact with the virus. Extra, booster vaccinations should be given if social contact and stress situations are unavoidable (e.g. boarding catteries, veterinary hospitals, or going to stud). Cattery owners should insist on recent vaccination and should take measures to keep the concentration of the virus in the environment to a minimum and to reduce contact between pens. Animals at particular risk (e.g. stud cats) should be boosted 6-monthly.

In virus-free colonies care should be taken to avoid buying in carriers; vaccinated animals may be free from disease but they are not necessarily free from infection. In breeding colonies where the disease is endemic, breeding queens should be regularly vaccinated, with additional boosters before mating, or during pregnancy if using a killed vaccine.

Kittening should be in isolation to keep kittens away from any carrier animals in the colony, and if it is likely that the queen herself is a carrier, then the kittens should be weaned early, at 4–5 weeks, and moved into a separate room. Kittens should be vaccinated as soon as maternal antibodies are at a non-interfering level (9 weeks is recommended by most manufacturers) and certainly before exposure to adult stock. In situations where it is not practical for kittens to be separated from their dams at an early age, earlier vaccination programmes may be initiated (e.g. starting at 5 or 6 weeks of age, and revaccinating at 3-week intervals until 12 weeks of age). Although not licensed for use in the UK in kittens less than 12 weeks of age, the early use of intranasal vaccination (e.g. starting at 3 weeks if disease is occurring in 4-week-old kittens) or a combination of both routes, may be helpful.

NASAL MYCOSES AND NEOPLASIA

Nasal mycoses and neoplasia are rare in the cat but should be considered in cases of refractory mucopurulent nasal discharge particularly where this is unilateral or associated with facial swelling. Lymphosarcoma may also involve the nasal cavities often as part of more widespread lymphosarcoma; such cases may well be negative on testing for FeLV viraemia. Diagnosis in these conditions is based on biopsy and histological examination of tissue. A biopsy sample can usually be obtained through the nares using biopsy forceps. The prognosis is guarded in nasal mycoses, though prolonged treatment with amphotericin B has been suggested. The prognosis is generally hopeless in cases of primary nasal carcinoma, though remission may be achieved in some cases of lymphosarcoma with cytotoxic or immunosuppressive drugs.

LOWER RESPIRATORY TRACT DISEASE

TRACHEAL DISEASE

Conditions affecting the trachea are uncommon in the cat. Tracheal collapse has been recorded but is rare except where associated with external compression, e.g. by anterior mediastinal lymphosarcoma. Tracheal foreign bodies may occur and occasionally upper respiratory tract virus infections may cause a tracheitis.

BRONCHIAL ASTHMA

Aetiology

The aetiology is unknown though it may be allergic.

Clinical signs and diagnosis

The condition is characterized by the sudden onset of paroxysmal, dry coughing and expiratory dyspnoea.

Radiographically the lung fields show a greater than normal radioluscency. Haematology reveals a marked eosinophilia (15–20%) in the majority of cases. Diagnosis, however, is based largely on response to treatment.

Treatment

The clinical signs respond to corticosteroid therapy, initially given intramuscularly (2 mg/kg bodyweight prednisolone) followed by oral dosage over about a week. The condition, however, tends to recur.

PNEUMONIA

Although pneumonia is uncommon in the cat, a primary viral pneumonia may be seen following infection with some FCV strains or as a complication of FVR. It may also be associated with inhalation of food following force feeding or persistent regurgitation, due for example to oesophageal strictures, vascular ring anomalies or megoesophagus, or occasionally with inhalation during medication with oily substances, such as liquid paraffin. Occasionally discrete pulmonary abscesses may form and more generalized pulmonary infections, e.g. fungal, tuberculosis, have also been recorded.

ALEUROSTRONGYLUS INFECTION

Clinical signs and diagnosis

Infection with the bronchiolar parasite *Aleurostrongylus abstruses* is often asymptomatic and self-limiting. In some cases heavy infestation may cause coughing and, rarely, secondary infection may lead to broncho-pneumonia. Diagnosis is based on the demonstration of first-stage larvae in the faeces or in bronchial washings. Small nodular densities may be seen on radiographic examination and haematological examination typically reveals a leucocytosis and an eosinophilia. Infection is rare in older cats.

Treatment

The treatment of choice is fenbendazole (Panacur, Hoechst) at a dose rate of 20 mg/kg bodyweight daily for 5 days.

PULMONARY NEOPLASIA

Primary pulmonary carcinoma in the cat leads to the accumulation of thoracic fluid and is discussed under diseases of the pleura. Involvement of the lung in multicentric neoplastic disease, e.g. lymphosarcoma, or metastatic disease, also occurs. Diagnosis is based on radiographic examination of the lung fields. Involvement is usually extensive before clinical signs of tachypnoea are appreciated.

PLEURAL DISEASE

Loss of thoracic capacity may be associated with a number of conditions (Table 2.2), cases of which invariably present as tachypnoea or dyspnoea particularly when the animal is stressed. Such cats require very gentle handling especially during radiography when only dorsoventral and erect lateral views may be possible. Ventrodorsal radiographs should not be attempted in the dyspnoeic cat as the position may cause fatal respiratory embarrassment.

RUPTURE OF THE DIAPHRAGM

Diagnosis

A history of recent trauma or the presence of other clinical signs indicating trauma such as skin abrasions, split claws or

Table 2.2 Pleural disease.

Rupture of the diaphragm
Pneumothorax
Haemothorax
Anterior mediastinal (thymic) lymphosarcoma
Exudative pleurisy
Chylothorax
Feline infectious peritonitis
Cardiomyopathy
Pulmonary carcinoma

bone fractures are helpful. Some cases of diaphragmatic rupture, however, especially those where liver incarceration in the chest leads to the formation of pleural fluid, may not become clinically apparent for weeks or even months. Auscultation of the chest may reveal areas of dullness and, more usefully, displacement of the heart sounds; borborygmi are unusual. The abdomen may feel empty on palpation. Elevation of the front part of the body may give some relief from the dyspnoea; the reverse, elevation of the rear end, is contraindicated.

Radiographs are invaluable in confirming a diagnosis (Figs. 2.4 and 2.5). The presence of fluid in the pleural cavity may mask radiographic evidence of a ruptured diaphragm. Such fluid, a blood-stained modified transudate, should be removed by thoracentesis and/or diuresis (e.g. frusemide) and the cat radiographed again.

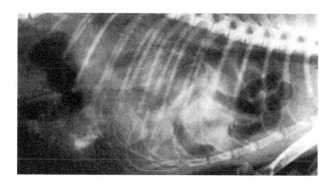

Fig. 2.4
Rupture of the diaphragm. Lateral chest radiograph showing gas- (or faecal-) filled bowel loops which have been displaced into the pleural cavity.

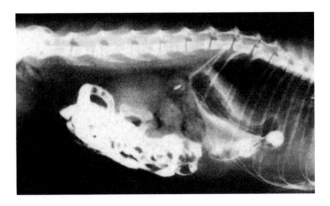

Fig. 2.5 Rupture of the diaphragm. Lateral radiograph taken following barium administration, showing cranial displacement of the stomach and, by inference, prolapse of the liver. Where the stomach or bowel cannot be readily identified or where tachypnoea makes a still radiograph impossible, a small (10 ml) administration of barium (Micropaque, Damancy Co Ltd) can be helpful.

Treatment

The replacement of abdominal organs in the peritoneal cavity and the repair of the diaphragmatic defect by surgical correction should be carried out as soon as practicable. Occasionally gastric prolapse and tympany may lead to a rapidly worsening dyspnoea and necessitate thoracentesis to relieve gastric distension, followed by surgical correction as soon as possible. The management of anaesthesia is critical, including rapid induction and introduction of an endotracheal tube to assist respiration; initiation of positive pressure anaesthesia when the peritoneal and hence the pleural cavity is entered; gradual reinflation of the lungs following replacement of abdominal organs; and reduction of pneumothorax during surgery or postoperatively.

PNEUMOTHORAX

Diagnosis

The presence of free air within the pleural cavity, which may follow a penetrating wound of the chest, rib fractures or spontaneous rupture of the lung following trauma, is best demonstrated radiographically (Fig 2.6). Penetration of the chest wall is usually associated with subcutaneous emphysema.

Treatment

The decision to aspirate the air rather than to wait for natural absorption depends on the condition and progress of the cat. Aspiration should be carried out in the dorsal third of the chest at about the seventh intercostal space and may need to be repeated. Indwelling pleural catheters, while possible, are rarely necessary.

HAEMOTHORAX

Diagnosis

Usually associated with trauma, the clinical signs of haemothorax may be due as much to hypovolaemia as to compression of lung tissue. The radiological appearance is that of any free fluid in the pleural cavity, though other evidence of trauma, e.g. fractured ribs, may also be present. Diagnosis is confirmed by the finding of blood on thoracentesis.

Treatment

Fluid therapy, warmth, or a blood transfusion, provide supportive treatment though rapid or continuous haemorrhage may necessitate exploratory thoracotomy.

ANTERIOR MEDIASTINAL (THYMIC) LYMPHOSARCOMA

Aetiology

A manifestation of feline leukaemia virus (FeLV) infection. The majority of cases of thymic lymphosarcoma are FeLV positive by virus isolation or ELISA.

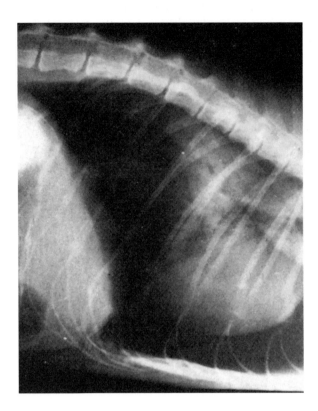

Fig. 2.6
Pneumothorax.
Lateral chest
radiograph showing
the "lifting" of the
apex of the heart
from the sternum by
an air density. In a
dorsoventral
projection free air is
seen lateral to the
lung lobes and
identified by the
failure of the lung
markings to extend to
the thoracic wall.

Clinical signs and diagnosis

Anterior mediastinal or thymic lymphosarcoma typically causes dyspnoea and regurgitation due to a mass compressing the trachea and oesophagus and to the formation of pleural fluid. Anorexia, depression and weight loss may also occur. On auscultation the heart sounds are displaced caudally and frequently muffled. Palpation of the cranial part of the chest reveals a marked reduction in the normal spring of the rib cage. This form of lymphosarcoma is typically seen in young cats, 8 months to 3 years, particularly of oriental breeds.

Approximately two-thirds of cases show evidence of a variable amount of pleural fluid. The diagnosis may be confirmed by radiography (Fig. 2.7) or, where fluid is present, by thoracentesis and by the demonstration on cytological examination of malignant lymphoblasts. The fluid is usually a clear or blood-stained modified transudate but occasional cases may be chylous.

Treatment

The prognosis is poor, though in some cases remission may be possible with cytotoxic and/or immunosuppressive therapy. The implications of FeLV infection for in-contact animals should be considered.

EXUDATIVE PLEURISY

Aetiology

The cause of exudative pleurisy (pyothorax or empyema) is not clear. Examination of the fluid usually reveals bacteria, though culture may be difficult and require aerobic and anaerobic techniques. Penetrating wounds of the chest, spread of subcutaneous infection and the extension of virus pneumonia have all been suggested though they are frequently absent in individual cases.

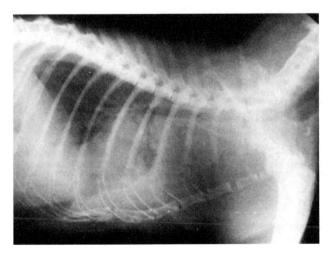

Fig. 2.7
Anterior mediastinal (thymic) lymphosarcoma. A lateral chest radiograph shows the normal radioluscency of the anterior mediastinum to be replaced by a soft tissue mass which displaces the trachea dorsally and the heart, the position of which is identified by the corina, caudally. Pleural fluid is also present.

Clinical signs and diagnosis

Cats with exudative pleurisy have tachypnoea and dyspnoea. They may also be pyrexic, depressed and inappetent. The onset of clinical signs may be quite sudden despite the apparent chronicity of the condition. Auscultation reveals thoracic dullness, particularly ventrally, and heart sounds are muffled.

Radiographs show the typical appearance of free fluid within the pleural cavity (Fig. 2.8). The fluid usually is bilateral but on occasions may be present only unilaterally. Diagnosis is confirmed by radiography and thoracentesis and the demonstration of an exudate which may vary in appearance from a reddish-brown watery fluid to a creamy-yellow inspissated material. Smears of the fluid reveal large numbers of leucocytes and Gram-stained smears usually show the presence of organisms.

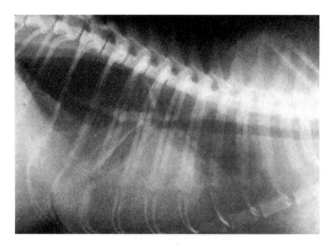

Fig. 2.8 Exudative pleurisy. Radiographs show typical appearance of free fluid in the pleural cavity. On this recumbent lateral view the dorsal borders of the diaphragmatic lung lobes are displaced ventrally from the thoracic vertebrae by a fluid density. Using a horizontal X-ray beam with the cat erect, fluid collects in the ventral portion of the chest where contrast is, therefore, lost. A dorso-ventral view shows displacement of the lungs by a fluid density from the lateral walls of the chest.

Treatment

Pleural fluid should be removed by thoracentesis and anti-biotics administered based on bacterial culture of the fluid and antibiotic sensitivity testing, though on occasions culture may not be successful. The prognosis is fair, though thoracentesis from both sides may be necessary and may have to be repeated on a number of occasions to achieve resolution. In rare cases, thoracotomy may be necessary to remove loculated or particularly thick pleural fluid. In cases refractory to treatment it may be advisable to check the animal's FeLV and FIV status.

CHYLOTHORAX

Aetiology

Trauma or neoplastic involvement of the thoracic duct.

Clinical signs and diagnosis

The main features are tachypnoea and subsequent dyspnoea. Radiographic examination of the chest reveals the presence of pleural fluid which may be identified as milky chyle on thoracentesis.

Treatment

Repeated drainage of the chyle, often over many weeks, may lead to resolution, presumably due to natural repair of the duct. Surgical repair of the duct has been described but is extremely difficult.

FELINE INFECTIOUS PERITONITIS (FIP)

Aetiology

Feline coronavirus. The majority of cases of "wet", typical or peritoneal FIP have ascites and although some 20% may also have pleural fluid this is rarely of clinical significance. In a very small number of cases, however, pleural fluid may predominate.

Clinical signs and diagnosis

Tachypnoea, dyspnoea with weight loss and inappetence occur in most cases. Following radiographic demonstration of fluid, thoracentesis reveals a characteristic straw coloured, tenacious fluid which clots on standing and is high in protein. The demonstration of high titres (> 1 in 320) of coronavirus antibody in both serum and pleural fluid may aid diagnosis, but such levels may be equivocal in some cases.

Treatment

Despite reports of limited success in treating FIP, the prognosis is invariably hopeless.

CARDIOMYOPATHY

Aetiology

An association between dilatory cardiomyopathy in cats and diets low in taurine has recently been established, and supplementation of commercial diets will probably lead to a reduction in incidence. Cardiomyopathy may also be associated with hyperthyroidism seen in older cats. Some cases of cardiomyopathy remain idiopathic.

Clinical signs and diagnosis

The congestive heart failure associated with cardiomyopathy in cats (Fig. 2.9) is characterized by pleural fluid and pulmonary oedema; this is appreciated clinically as tachypnoea and dyspnoea. Heart rate is rapid (200 +) and ectopic heart beats may be seen on an electrocardiogram. The fluid is a watery "modified" transudate. Cardiomyopathy in cats is also associated with the development of aortic emboli and the sudden onset of posterior paralysis with absence of femoral pulse, spasm of the gastrocnemius muscles and coldness of the hind limbs.

Treatment

Diuretic treatment of the congestive heart failure (e.g. frusemide) may give a temporary improvement. Cardiac glycosides are poorly tolerated by cats and are not generally helpful. The use of vasodilators, e.g. captopril, has yet to be fully evaluated in cats but may be helpful. The long term prognosis is grave.

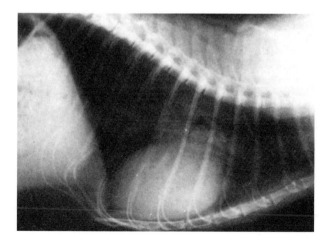

Fig. 2.9
Cardiomyopathy.
Lateral chest
radiograph made
following the removal
of fluid by diuresis
showing
cardiomegally.

PULMONARY CARCINOMA

Aetiology

Unknown.

Clinical signs and diagnosis

Pulmonary carcinoma is seen in older cats and causes
tachypnoea and dyspnoea due to the accumulation of pleural
fluid. Diagnosis is based on radiographic signs (Fig. 2.10),
the demonstration of a modified transudate on thoracentesis
and, if necessary, the findings at exploratory thoracotomy.

Treatment

None. Diuresis may provide temporary relief.

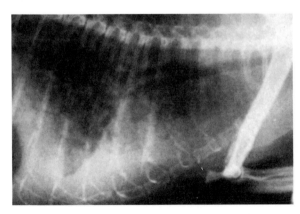

Fig. 2.10
Pulmonary carcinoma. Lateral
chest radiograph showing
pleural fluid and mottled
increased radiodensities
throughout the lung fields.

FURTHER READING

UPPER RESPIRATORY TRACT DISEASE

Gaskell, R. M. (1981). In *The Veterinary Annual*, 21st Issue (eds C. S. Grunsell & F. W. G. Hill), pp. 267–274, Scientechnica, Bristol. An assessment of the use of feline respiratory virus vaccines.

Gaskell, R. M. (1985). Viral-induced respiratory disease. In *Feline Medicine and Therapeutics* (eds E. A. Chandler, C. J. Gaskell & A. D. R. Hilberry) pp. 257–270. Blackwell, Oxford.

Gaskell, R. M. (1988). Feline respiratory disease complex. In *Manual of Small Animal Infectious Diseases* (ed J. E. Barlough) pp. 119–135. Churchill Livingstone, New York.

Gaskell, R. M. (1990). *Journal of Small Animal Practice* **30**, 618–624.

Lane, J. G. (1977). In *The Veterinary Annual*, 17th issue (eds C. S. Grunsell & F. W. G. Hill) pp. 164–168. Wright-Scientechnica, Bristol. Pharyngostomy intubation of the dog and cat.

Povey, R. C. (1990). Feline respiratory disease. In *Infectious Diseases of the Dog and Cat* (ed. C. E. Greene) pp. 346–357. W. B. Saunders, Philadelphia.

PLEURAL DISEASE

Gruffydd-Jones, T. J. & Flecknell, P. A. (1978). *Journal of Small Animal Practice* **19**, 315–328. The prognosis and treatment related to the gross appearance and laboratory characteristics of pathological thoracic fluids in the cat.

Gruffydd-Jones, T. J., Gaskell, C. J. & Gibbs, C. (1979). *Veterinary Record* **104**, 304–307. Clinical and radiological features of anterior mediastinal lymphosarcoma in the cat: a review of 30 cases.

Squires, R. A. & Gorman N. T. (1990). Antineoplastic chemotherapy in cats. *In Practice* **12**(3), 101–111.

CHAPTER 3

Upper Respiratory Tract Diseases

ROSALIND GASKELL AND JONATHAN KNOWLES

INTRODUCTION

Despite the advent of vaccination in the mid-1970s, infectious respiratory disease in cats still occurs, although vaccination has probably reduced the overall severity of the condition.

AETIOLOGY

The causes of infectious respiratory disease in cats together with an estimate of their significance are listed in Table 3.1.

Feline viral rhinotracheitis (FVR) virus, also known as felid herpesvirus 1 (FHV 1), and feline calicivirus (FCV) are the two major causes of respiratory disease in cats. Both are widespread in the cat population and have generally been considered to be of equal importance. Recently, however, we have observed a slightly higher isolation rate of FCV than expected compared to FHV 1. This may be explained in part by the antigenic diversity among FCV isolates and the consequent relative efficacy of each of the two vaccines.

Recently feline *Chlamydia psittaci* has been identified in the UK as a significant cause of disease where the predominant

Table 3.1 Causes and significance of infectious respiratory disease in the cat.

Agents	Significance
Feline viral rhinotracheitis virus (felid herpesvirus 1)	Approximately 40% of cases. Tends to be more severe
Feline calicivirus	Approximately 40% of cases, possibly more. Usually mild
Feline *Chlamydia psittaci*	Approximately 30% of cases of persistent conjunctivitis
Feline reovirus	Mild disease experimentally. Significance in the field unknown
Feline poxvirus	Occasional respiratory/ ocular signs but other, skin signs also present
Feline infectious peritonitis virus (feline coronavirus)	Most likely a primary, enteric pathogen, but respiratory signs also suggested by some
Bordetella species	Some laboratory colonies. Clinically significant?
Other bacteria e.g. *Staphlococcus, Streptococcus and Pasteurellae* species; coliforms	Mainly secondary invaders
Mycoplasmas	Possibly primary, mainly secondary infection

clinical sign is a persistent conjunctivitis. Feline reovirus has long been cited as a possible cause of mild conjunctival and respiratory disease in cats, on the basis of some limited experimental work in the USA some years ago. Its importance in the field has never been established. In recent virological studies undertaken specifically for reovirus, we found no evidence of this infection in over 150 conjunctival samples from cats with conjunctivitis.

Other agents, with only suspected or peripheral involvement with feline respiratory disease are listed in Table 3.1. Bacteria and mycoplasmas are mainly important as secondary invaders.

Finally, the pathogenicity of all agents, including secondary invaders, may be enhanced as a result of concurrent illness especially immunosuppressive (e.g. infection with feline leukaemia virus (FeLV) or, the newly recognized feline immunodeficiency virus (FIV).

CLINICAL SIGNS

A brief summary of the essential clinical features of the three major conditions, namely FVR, FCV infection, and *C. psittaci* infection, is shown in Table 3.2.

Although there is considerable overlap between the diseases, some distinction may be drawn from the predominant clinical signs. Thus a more severe syndrome, with copious ocular and nasal discharges, might suggest FVR. If milder upper respiratory and ocular signs are present however and, especially if there is also ulceration of the tongue, hard palate, or external nares, then it is more likely to be FCV. A febrile "limping" syndrome also has been noted to occur with FCV. For both these diseases, milder signs will generally be seen in cats which have been vaccinated. If the major presenting clinical sign is persistent or recurrent conjunctivitis, then *C. psittaci* infection should be considered, especially in colonies that have been fully vaccinated against the respiratory viruses.

Recent work has shown that a high percentage of cats with chronic stomatitis and gingivitis are persistently infected with FCV, and a high proportion of such animals also have antibody to FIV.

DIAGNOSIS

To some extent a diagnosis may be made on presenting clinical signs, but where a definitive diagnosis is required, confirmatory laboratory tests are necessary. For the respiratory viruses, an oropharyngeal swab should be taken, placed in viral transport medium and sent first class post to a laboratory for attempted virus isolation.

For chlamydia, although conjunctival scrapings may be examined directly for the presence of inclusion bodies, a more reliable diagnosis may be made from a vigorous conjunctival swab sent in special transport medium to an appropriate laboratory for attempted isolation of the organism, or possibly testing by ELISA.

Serology is generally not helpful for the respiratory viruses, because of widespread immunity from vaccination, but it may be helpful in establishing a possible diagnosis of C. *psittaci* infection.

TREATMENT

Treatment has been described in more detail elsewhere (Gaskell, 1985). In viral respiratory disease, the main emphasis should be on adequate antibiotic treatment to counter secondary bacterial infection, with fluid therapy in more severe cases

Table 3.2 Comparison of the relative importance of individual clinical signs seen in the major respiratory infections of cats.

Clinical signs	Feline viral rhinotracheitis	Feline calicivirus infection*	Feline *Chlamydia psittaci* infection
General malaise	+ + +	+	+
Sneezing	+ + +	+	+
Hypersalivation	+ +	+/−	−
Conjunctivitis	+ +	+ +	+ + +**
Ocular discharge	+ + +	+ +	+ + +
Nasal discharge	+ + +	+ +	+
Oral ulceration	+	+ + +	−
Keratitis	+	−	−
Primary pneumonia	(+)	+	+/−
Limping	−	+	+

*   Strain variation occurs.
**   Often persistent.
(+) Rare, but has been reported.
+/− Signs may be present, but not usually obvious clinically.

where dehydration may become a problem. Good nursing can make an important contribution to recovery.

Corticosteroids are contraindicated because they may potentiate the virus infection. At present no anti-viral drugs are in widespread use. However, IUdR has been used in ulcerative keratitis in FVR, and there are other anti-herpesvirus drugs developed for use in other species which may prove useful in this disease.

In *C. psittaci* infection, although several antibiotics may have some effect on the organism, the antibiotic of choice is oxytetracycline. As the organism may generalize throughout the body systemic treatment should be given in addition to local. Treatment should also be continued for at least four weeks, or two weeks after clinical signs have disappeared, because eradication can be difficult.

EPIZOOTIOLOGY

FELINE RESPIRATORY VIRUSES

Both FHV 1 and FCV are highly successful pathogens of the cat, although infection is more common in colony animals than in individual household pets. Thus the disease occurs mainly in boarding catteries, breeding colonies, stray cat homes, or other situations where large numbers of cats have been brought together.

The feline respiratory viruses persist in the cat population in three main ways (Figure 3.1).

(1) By passing directly from acutely infected to susceptible animals. This depends on the presence of a sufficient number of susceptible animals in the population and sufficient opportunities for contact between them.
(2) By persisting in the environment. Although this is for only relatively short periods of time, it is nevertheless long enough for indirect transmission to occur, particularly within the close confines of a cattery: aerosol transmission is not thought to be of major significance.
(3) By persisting in the recovered cat as a carrier state. Despite vaccination, our recent figures indicate that such

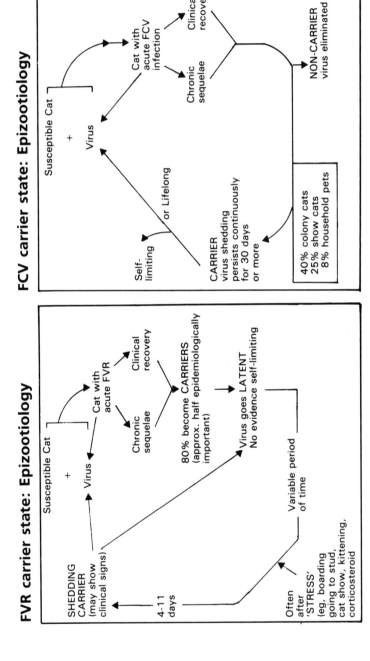

Fig. 3.1 A diagrammatic representation of the major features of the carrier states for both FVR and FCV infections.

carriers still seem to be widespread in the population and are of considerable importance as a source of virus.

There are no known reservoir hosts for the viruses, and vertical transmission does not seem to occur.

FELINE *C. PSITTACI* INFECTION

Although many species of animals and birds are susceptible to *C. psittaci* infection, there are a variety of strains of the organism of different tropisms, pathogenicity, and host specificity. Although some are zoonotic, the feline strain generally appears to be species specific. Like the feline respiratory viruses, chlamydial infection is probably transmitted mainly by direct or fomite contact with infectious discharges from acutely or chronically infected cats; clinical signs may persist or recur for some time, and shedding may persist for several months. The organism is found mainly in ocular secretions, but vaginal and rectal shedding has also been recorded in experimentally infected cats; the epidemiological significance of this is unknown.

PREVENTION AND CONTROL

VIRAL RESPIRATORY DISEASES

The prevention and control of viral respiratory disease in different cat populations has been described in detail by Gaskell (1985). Completely successful control of these diseases may, however, be difficult, particularly in certain situations. Although vaccination can be reasonably effective in providing protection, the nature of the epizootiology of the disease means that control is best attempted through a combination of vaccination and management. Where problems associated with vaccination occur, they fall broadly into two categories – vaccine reactions and vaccine breakdowns.

Vaccine reactions

The most likely cause for this is that the cat is already incubating the disease at the time of vaccination: most vaccination programmes are implemented in kittens at the time that their maternal antibody wanes.

It is possible that an older cat is already a carrier: in FVR, this could mean that the mild disruption of the cat's normal routine by vaccination may initiate an episode of viral recrudescence with clinical signs. Modified live vaccines should be attenuated so as not to cause disease; however, some individuals may be immunologically incompetent, perhaps because of intercurrent disease, or they may have different microbial flora. Even in apparently normal cats, however, intranasal vaccines may cause some clinical signs, but this can be offset in some situations by the advantage that they can induce a more rapid immunity. In contrast, live parenteral vaccines should be safe, but if they inadvertently reach the respiratory mucosa, they too may induce clinical signs. Recently, the use of live vaccines has occasionally been associated with a "limping" syndrome, seen most commonly following primary vaccination. In some cases, this may be attributable to the calicivirus component of the vaccine, but in most instances it is probably due to a coincidental field virus infection.

Vaccine breakdowns

First, although the respiratory vaccines are reasonably effective, it should be emphasized that, even under ideal conditions, protection is not necessarily complete. In less than ideal conditions, intercurrent disease, especially with the immunodeficiency viruses, an overwhelming dose of challenge virus, or maternal (passive) antibody interference may adversely affect protection conferred by vaccines.

In colonies with enzootic disease, breakdowns may be fairly common. Maternal antibody protection may be of short and variable duration and thus disease tends to occur in young kittens. Carriers are widespread in such colonies, ensuring a continuous supply of challenge virus. Furthermore, vaccination does not eliminate infection from cats that are already carriers, and a previously unexposed, vaccinated cat can subsequently become infected subclinically and become a field virus carrier under cover of vaccine immunity.

It is also apparent that the present widely used FCV vaccine strain does not protect against all isolates of the virus, and future vaccines may need to incorporate several complementary, cross-protective isolates. Finally, in apparent vaccine breakdowns infection may be caused by agents not included in the vaccine, such as *C. psittaci*.

CHLAMYDIAL INFECTION

The prevention and control of chlamydial infection should be approached both by good management, and by the effective use of antibiotics. Because persistent or recurrent infection is common, all cats in a colony should be treated at the same time. Although vaccination has been employed against *C. psittaci* in the USA for some time, there is no vaccine currently available in the UK. Although there has been discussion as to the efficacy of such vaccines, recent studies have indicated some protection against the disease, although not necessarily against shedding of the organism.

REFERENCES AND FURTHER READING

Gaskell, R. M. (1981). An assessment of the use of feline respiratory virus vaccines. *The Veterinary Annual* 21st issue (eds C. S. G. Grunsell & F. W. G. Hill) pp. 267–274. Scientechnica, Bristol.

Gaskell, R. M. (1985). Viral-induced respiratory disease. In *Feline Medicine and Therapeutics* (eds E. A. Chandler, C. J. Gaskell & A. D. R. Hilbery), pp. 257–270. Blackwells, Oxford.

Gaskell, R. M. (1988). Feline respiratory disease complex. In *Manual of Small Animal Infectious Diseases* (ed. J. E. Barlough), pp. 119–135. Churchill Livingstone, New York.

Gaskell, R. M. (1990). Vaccination of the young kitten. *Journal of Small Animal Practice* **30**, 618–624.

Povey, R. C. (1990). Feline respiratory disease. In *Infectious Diseases of the Dog and Cat* (ed. C. E. Greene), pp. 346–357. W. B. Saunders, Philadelphia.

CHAPTER 4

Differential Diagnosis of Dyspnoea

ALISON BLAXTER

INTRODUCTION

Dyspnoea is a common presenting sign in cats and may often be the only indication of thoracic disease. It is one of the most common reasons for referral of cats to Bristol University. The characteristic posture associated with dyspnoea is sternal recumbency, with flexed, abducted elbows. Obvious tachypnoea and hyperpnoea are often accompanied by coughing and abnormal respiratory noise. Gross exercise intolerance is rare. Cats readily adopt less strenuous lifestyles and in a non-debilitated dyspnoeic cat, weight gain may even be a noticeable sign.

For ease of discussion causes of dyspnoea can be listed as in Table 4.1; however, divisions may be arbitrary when considering a specific condition.

INVESTIGATION OF DYSPNOEA

HISTORY

Historical features may help identify the aetiology of dyspnoea. For example, cases of tracheal or bronchial foreign bodies are usually acute in onset, may result in bouts of cyanosis, coughing, respiratory noise and effort and may eventually be accompanied by noticeable halitosis. A history of trauma, such as a road traffic accident, may suggest dyspnoea to be a result of ruptured diaphragm or a traumatic pleural effusion.

GENERAL CLINICAL EXAMINATION

Most information comes from detailed examination of the thorax and upper respiratory tract but a general physical examination may sometimes suggest an aetiology or line of investigation. For example, profound weight loss and wasting in an older dyspnoeic cat might suggest hyperthyroidism with secondary cardiomyopathy. Stunting in a young cat may prompt suspicion of a congenital cardiac anomaly. The general demeanour of a systemically ill, pyrexic or depressed cat may indicate dyspnoea to be but one feature of a multisystemic or infective disorder.

Examination of the mouth and mucous membranes may reveal features of upper respiratory virus infection with ulcerations being prominent in infection with feline calici virus. Cyanosis (Fig. 4.1) is a feature of right to left vascular shunts (such as tetralogy of Fallot) and can accompany the severe airway obstruction of tracheal collapse and inhaled foreign bodies.

Examination of the cervical area and thoracic inlet may be useful in some cases. Hyperthyroidism causes secondary hypertrophic cardiomyopathy and is associated with functioning thyroid neoplasms which are often palpable just below the larynx. In other cases palpation of the thoracic inlet may suggest lack of normal compliance because of a cranial intrathoracic mass.

Examination of the abdomen may be relevant. Ascitic fluid is usually present in the effusive form of feline infectious

Table 4.1 Causes of dyspnoea.

Upper airway obstruction

Nasal and pharyngeal disease	Viral infections
	Nasopharyngeal polyps
	Neoplasia
	Foreign bodies
	Mycotic infections

Laryngeal disease	Neoplasia
	Paralysis

Lower airway obstruction

Tracheal diseases	Collapse
	Stenosis
	Foreign body
	External compression
	Neoplasia

Bronchial disease	Parasitic bronchitis
	Eosinophilic bronchitis (feline asthma)

Pulmonary disease

Primary pulmonary carcinoma
Pneumonia/bronchopneumonia
Pulmonary abcessation
Poisoning, e.g., paraquat, ANTU, paracetamol
Oedema
Haemorrhage

Disorders of the thoracic cavity

Pleural effusions	Feline infectious peritonitis
	Exudative pleurisy
	Traumatic – haemothorax, chylothorax, pneumothorax
	Congestive heart failure
	Lung lobe torsion
	Nephrotic syndrome

Thoracic masses	Thymic lymphosarcoma
	Diaphragmatic rupture
	Pericardioperitoneal diaphragmatic hernia

Cardiac disease

Congenital anomalies
Cardiomyopathy – primary and secondary
Congestive heart failure (as a result of the above)

Physiological

Fear, pain, shock, anaemia, pyrexia

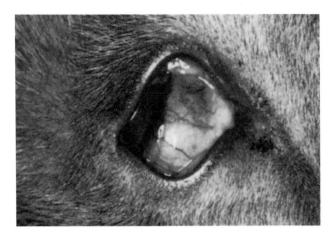

Fig. 4.1
Cyanosis is an
uncommon but
dramatic presenting
feature in the
dyspnoeic cat and is
a prominent clinical
sign in right to left
cardiac shunt and in
severe obstruction of
the lower airways.

peritonitis; hepatomegaly can occur in congestive heart failure and diaphragmatic rupture may result in an empty feel on abdominal palpation.

Detailed examination of the respiratory tract includes the upper airways. Obstructive upper airway disease will be accompanied by inspiratory noise and effort, while expiratory effort and noise derive from the lower respiratory tract. Nasal and ocular discharges are features of "cat flu", and nasal discharge with epistaxis and facial distortion are prominent signs in nasal neoplasia. Examination of the external ear canal and questioning as to aural discharge may be relevant in considering upper airway dyspnoea due to obstructive naso-pharyngeal polyps.

CLINICAL EXAMINATION OF THE THORAX

Palpation of the thoracic wall

Palpation of the thoracic wall may reveal gross deformity such as that found in flat-chested kittens, reduced chest compliance associated with thymic lymphosarcoma or the more subtle appreciation of a thrill associated with severe (usually congenital) cardiac abnormalities.

Percussion

The cat's chest wall presents only a small area for percussion and may be unrewarding. Dullness is sometimes a dramatic indication of a mass effusion, while pneumothorax produces areas of increased resonance.

Auscultation

Auscultation is very useful in the assessment of dyspnoea. Gross cardiomegaly, displacement or muffling of heart sounds, cardiac murmurs, gallop sounds, tachycardia, arrhythmias or adventitious lung sounds may be audible.

FURTHER INVESTIGATION

Radiography

Radiography is the most useful aid to clinical examination (Table 4.2) but has to be performed with care in a dyspnoeic patient. A right recumbent lateral view of the thorax that includes the anterior abdomen is probably the most useful projection although if there is pleural effusion or severe dyspnoea a dorsoventral view may be appropriate. These are best performed with the cat in a foam rubber trough to aid positioning and reduce stress.

Radiography of the upper respiratory tract is also a useful method of investigation of obstructive dyspnoea although it may not be the first approach and usually requires general anaesthesia. If a nasopharyngeal polyp is suspected, lateral

Table 4.2 Features assessable from thoracic radiographs.

Cardiac size, shape and position
Integrity of the diaphragm
Pulmonary fields – area, infiltrations
Effusions – fluid
Displacement of thoracic organs by masses
Patency of trachea and major bronchi

views may demonstrate a mass above or behind the soft palate and space occupying lesions outside the airways may displace and restrict the larynx or trachea. Intra-oral views of the nasal cavity are the best way to assess conditions confined to the nasal chambers.

Fluoroscopy

Fluoroscopy may be the only way to confirm episodic tracheal collapse, although still films of a suspected tracheal collapse taken while the animal is dyspnoeic and on inspiration may suggest the condition.

Angiography

Angiography may be useful in confirming and identifying gross congenital cardiac anomalies. Non-selective angiograms can occasionally assist in identifying left to right shunting but otherwise selective angiography with cardiac catheterization is necessary.

Electrocardiography

Cats with cardiomyopathy or congenital cardiac anomalies will commonly display abnormalities on ECG. These include increased height and width of QRS complexes, notching and widening of P waves, dysrhythmias, tachycardia (greater than 200 beats per minute) and abnormalities in conduction.

Thoracentesis

If pleural effusion is present, thoracentesis is useful in diagnosis and in treatment. Examination of the fluid allows assessment of aetiology (Table 4.3). Thoracic drainage may also allow the heart or a thoracic mass to be seen on X-ray. Thoracentesis is best performed on the right side (in bilateral effusions) at the seventh or eighth rib space, a third of the way up the chest wall with the cat in sternal recumbency.

Table 4.3 Investigation of pleural fluid in the cat.

	Gross appearance	Globulin content (g/litre)	Cytology	Bacterial culture
Feline infectious peritonitis	Yellow-tinged, tacky, may clot on standing, occasionally blood stained. Occasionally pseudochylous if long standing	> 40	Non-specific	Negative
Exudative pleurisy	Purulent-opaque, creamy yellow. Occasionally blood stained or with a green tinge. Flocculent	< 10	Large numbers of white blood cells predominantly neutrophils	Positive in most cases
Thymic lymphosarcoma	Clear, chylous or blood tinged	< 10	Variable number of lymphocytes and immature blast cells	Negative
Ruptured diagphragm/dia-phragmatic hernia	Clear or blood tinged	< 5	Non-specific	Negative
Congestive heart failure	Clear or blood tinged	< 5	Small numbers of neutrophils lymphocytes and reticulo endothelial cells	Negative
Pulmonary carcinoma	Clear or blood tinged	< 10	Small numbers of neutrophils and endothelial cells	Negative

Radiographs should be taken before this procedure to ensure that this site will provide fluid drainage, especially in a one-sided effusion.

The area should first be clipped and prepared aseptically, local anaesthetic infused under the skin and then a needle or catheter with a three-way tap introduced. The types of fluid and their features are outlined in the table. It is vital that these be considered in conjunction with clinical findings and radiographic examinations before and after thoracentesis. For example, feline infectious peritonitis may also produce ascitic fluid, pulmonary carcinoma will be evident as multiple opacities in the lung fields and a thymic lymphosarcoma will be visible as a mass displacing heart and trachea in the anterior thorax.

Bronchoscopy

If a tracheal or laryngeal disorder is suspected, bronchoscopy may aid diagnosis. Examination of bronchial washings retrieved after flushing the trachea with 20–30 ml of sterile saline may suggest disease such as eosinophilic or parasitic bronchitis.

Laboratory tests

Routine haematology may suggest or substantiate a diagnosis. In bronchial asthma there may be a circulating eosinophilia; feline infectious peritonitis can produce non-regenerative anaemia with lymphopenia and neutrophilia. Infective bacterial conditions such as bronchopneumonia, chronic rhinitis and exudative pleurisy may show a leucocytosis with neutrophilia and left shift.

Serum biochemistry is not of general value in the investigation of dyspnoea, but hyperglobulinaemia is a striking feature of feline infectious peritonitis and acute hepatocellular damage may be evident in hyperthyroidism. Severe hypoalbuminaemia rarely induces thoracic transudate in the cat.

Recovery of virus from the oropharynx may help confirm the cause of upper respiratory obstructive disease and serological examination for antibodies to the coronavirus of feline infectious peritonitis and feline leukaemia virus may be useful.

Aerobic and anaerobic culture of intrathoracic fluid is necessary to select the most appropriate treatment for exudative pleurisy and cytological examination of these fluids, and of tracheal or bronchial washings may be of use.

SPECIFIC CONDITIONS

DYSPNOEA DUE TO AIRWAY OBSTRUCTION

Upper airway (Table 4.4)

Chronic rhinitis

Feline calici virus and feline viral rhinotracheitis are causes of upper respiratory tract infection in the cat. These often result in chronic bacterial rhinitis with persistent bilateral mucopurulent discharge. Obstruction of the nasal chambers results and secondary sinusitis may develop. Virus may be recovered from oropharyngeal swabs. Intra-oral radiographs will demonstrate generalized loss of lucency in nasal cavities and lateral views may demonstrate soft tissue density in the frontal sinuses.

Nasal neoplasia

Both feline leukaemia virus associated lymphosarcoma and squamous cell carcinoma can involve the nasal cavities of the older cat and result in unilateral then bilateral discharge, epistaxis and facial distortion. Radiographs will suggest turbinate destruction (Fig. 4.2) and transnasal biopsy by needle or suction can confirm the diagnosis although exploratory rhinotomy may be necessary.

Nasopharyngeal polyps

Inflammatory polyps may arise from either the middle ear or eustachian tube and are fleshy, benign masses that can occlude nasal chambers, pharynx or external ear canals. They occur most commonly in young cats and there may be a history of upper respiratory viral infection. Otorrhoea, otitis interna, bilateral mucopurulent nasal discharge, upper respiratory obstructive dyspnoea and dysphagia are common signs. Diagnosis is confirmed by lateral radiographs of the pharynx and examination of external ear canals and pharynx under general anaesthesia.

Nasal aspergillosis and cryptococcosis

Although rare cases of nasal disease in the cat, these have been reported. Most commonly they induce unilateral nasal discharge and are not common causes of obstructive dyspnoea. Diagnosis can be confirmed by radiographic, microbiological, microscopic, serological and histological examinations.

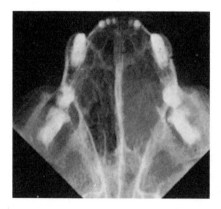

Fig. 4.2
In nasal neoplasia there is often striking unilateral loss of turbinate structure with a general increase in radio-opacity in the affected side. Septal deviation and rupture are also common features.

Foreign body rhinitis

Foreign bodies can cause destructive rhinitis and may be difficult, if radiolucent, to differentiate from nasal neoplasia and nasal mycosis. Exploratory rhinotomy may be advisable.

Lower airway

Larynx

The cat's larynx is the site for several disease processes that are often overlooked. Lymphosarcoma of the larynx or of surrounding tissues results in acute obstructive dyspnoea with stridor, a high pitched inspiratory wheeze and dramatic inspiratory effort. Laryngeal paralysis is not common in the cat and has been associated with lymphosarcomatous infiltration. However, idiopathic unilateral and bilateral paralysis is being increasingly recognized in young cats (between 1 and 3 years of age) and the inspiratory dyspnoea in such cases can be intermittent and exacerbated by stress. Laryngeal foreign bodies are uncommon causes of dyspnoea.

Trachea

Expiratory dyspnoea has been recorded in cases of intratracheal neoplasia and compression of the trachea by neoplastic masses in the cervical region or mediastinum. Intermittent tracheal collapse may also result in obstructive dyspnoea (Fig. 4.3). Tracheal and less commonly bronchial foreign bodies are a more common cause of dyspnoea in the cat (Fig. 4.4). The dyspnoea is often dramatic in onset, the clinical history involving a return from the garden in a cyanotic and dyspnoeic state. Coughing and expiratory noise are also features. The foreign body may cause incomplete occlusion of the airway and intermittent dyspnoea results, often progressing to halitosis and bronchopneumonia. Radiographic diagnosis is possible in those foreign bodies that are radio-opaque and other findings may suggest radiolucent foreign bodies. Endoscopy is usually necessary for diagnosis and treatment (Fig. 4.5).

Table 4.4 Radiographic and clinical differentiation of upper airway dyspnoea.

	Clinical/laboratory features	Radiography	
		Intra-oral view	Lateral skull/pharynx
Chronic viral rhinitis	Bilateral mucopurulent nasal discharge, recurrent ocular discharge, conjunctivitis, oral ulceration. Virus often recovered from oropharynx	Bilateral loss of radiolucency in nasal chambers with intact nasal turbinates	Soft tissue filling of frontal sinuses
Destructive rhinitis in nasal mycosis/foreign body	Persistent unilateral nasal discharge. Occasionally epistaxis and facial distortion. Bacteriology and histology demonstrate fungal infection	Unilateral destruction of nasal turbinates with patchy decrease in radio-opacity, in the most severely affected side. Uncommonly bilateral	Facial distortion possible but uncommon
Nasopharyngeal polyps	Bilateral or unilateral mucopurulent nasal discharge with dysphagia and often otitis externa or interna in a young cat	Non-specific	Soft tissue mass in nasopharyngeal air space. Ventral compression of the soft palate is common
Nasal neoplasia	Nasal discharge often unilateral, particularly initially, epistaxis, facial distortion in an older cat	Loss of turbinate pattern with variable changes in radio-opacity but usually a generalized increase, septal deviation possible, often unilateral	Occasionally evidence of facial distortion

Bronchial conditions

Bronchial disease although not uncommon in the cat is not well understood and may induce coughing rather than

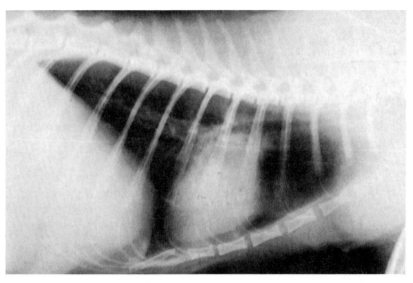

Fig. 4.3 Tracheal collapse is an uncommon but striking cause of lower airway obstruction in the cat. The most common site for collapse appears to be the thoracic inlet and in the case shown an area of collapse is seen at ribs 1 and 2.

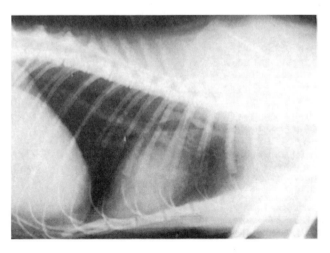

Fig. 4.4
Tracheal foreign bodies may appear as opaque densities in the airway.

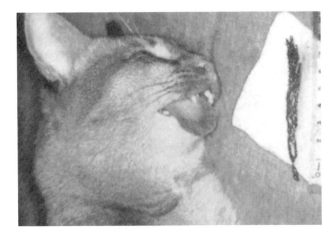

Fig. 4.5
Other tracheal foreign
bodies are not radio-
dense and may be
seen only by
bronchoscopy under
general anaesthetic.

dyspnoea. Bronchopneumonia is most common in young
kittens where low body temperatures allow colonization of the
lower respiratory tract, or can occur in an immunosuppressed
animal (for example in feline leukaemia virus infection).

Parasitic bronchitis

Parasitic bronchitis is recognized in the cat but many cats
may be infested with *Aleurostrongylus abstrusus* without clinical
signs. Coughing is the most prominent feature: the disorder
usually resolves without treatment.

Eosinophilic bronchitis (feline asthma)

Eosinophilic bronchitis is a poorly defined condition of chronic
bronchitis in the cat. The similarity to human allergic asthmatic
disease in clinical presentation, radiographic findings, eosinophilic tracheo-bronchial exudate and circulating eosinophilia
suggests that allergy is involved, although allergens have
rarely been identified. Cats are presented with recurrent
attacks of dyspnoea, paroxysmal coughing, wheezing and
expiratory effort. Attacks can be severe enough to induce
gasping and cyanosis. Patchy, non-specific infiltration of lung
parenchyma is found radiographically; between 50 and 75%

of cases have a circulating eosinophilia and the response to corticosteroids is often dramatic.

PULMONARY CONDITIONS

Primary pulmonary carcinoma

Primary pulmonary carcinoma is a relatively common neoplasm of the older cat (Fig. 4.6) and characteristically induces pleural effusion, dyspnoea and an unproductive cough. Although the condition is usually insidious in its development in causing weight loss, the onset of signs can be acute and often without signs of debilitation. Radiographically, pulmonary carcinoma is visible as discrete masses or as diffuse dense infiltrations of the lung fields although these are often initially masked by pleural fluid. Examination of fluid obtained by thoracentesis demonstrates a clear, occasionally blood-tinged, modified transudate. Cytological examination very occasionally reveals neoplastic cells but findings are usually non-specific. If a diagnosis cannot be made from radiography and cytology, percutaneous biopsy is possible. If necessary, exploratory thoracotomy will confirm the diagnosis.

Pneumonia and bronchopneumonia

These are rare in the adult cat and often sequelae to immunosuppressive disease. They are also more commonly causes of

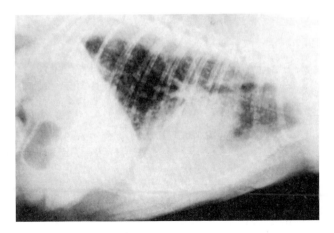

Fig. 4.6
Primary pulmonary
carcinoma in the cat
results in patchy
infiltration in the lung
fields of older,
dyspnoeic cats.

coughing rather than dyspnoea. Infections with toxoplasma or pox virus are possible causes.

Pulmonary abcessation

Discrete abcessation in pulmonary tissue can cause intermittent dyspnoea with pyrexia, depression and anorexia. These areas will be visible on radiographs and percutaneous aspiration of the areas for bacteriological examination is possible. They may be the result of traumatic puncture wounds to the chest, but in most cases the aetiology is unknown.

Right diaphragmatic lobar pneumonia is often caused by an inhaled foreign body.

DISORDERS OF THE THORACIC CAVITY

Pleural effusion

Dyspnoea is the major clinical sign associated with pleural effusion. On auscultation there is usually muffling of heart sounds and lung sounds may be confined to a small area of the dorsal thorax. Percussion may suggest a fluid line with areas of dullness and radiographs will demonstrate the presence of fluid as an increase in soft tissue density obscuring detail of the ventral thorax (Fig. 4.7). Lung lobes will be collapsed. Thoracentesis is the main aid to diagnosis and treatment.

Exudative pleurisy (pyothorax or empyaemia)

Chronic accumulations of infected fluids in the chest are common in the cat. Often the source of infection remains unknown but pyothorax can follow puncture wounds of the thoracic cavity, and haematogenous spread from infected foci at distant sites is also thought to occur. The clinical signs may include an intermittent pyrexia but often the cat is presented in acute dyspnoea. After thoracentesis of purulent, often foul-smelling fluid, radiography may demonstrate rounded caudal lung lobes and pockets of remaining fluid. Bacterial examin-

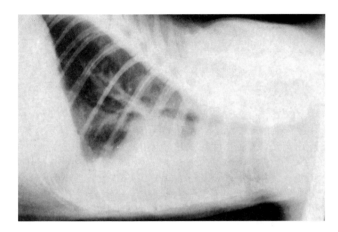

Fig. 4.7
Pleural effusion
results in soft tissue
density obscuring
detail of the ventral
thorax.

ation of the fluid often reveals a range of aerobic and anaerobic organisms. The prognosis of these cases must be guarded but between 50 and 75% of cases respond fully to treatment.

Feline infectious peritonitis

The "effusive" or "wet" form of feline infectious peritonitis characteristically induces ascites but 20% of these cases will also have pleural effusion and be presented with dyspnoea. Occasionally pleural effusion alone will be a presenting feature. Classically the fluid is bilateral, yellow, thick and tacky with a high globulin content and hyperglobulineamia is found. Occasionally pseudochylous effusions (lactescent fluids that are not ether-soluble) are found if the fluid is long standing.

Diagnosis is based on the clinical signs which may include persistent intermittent pyrexia, ascites, jaundice, non-regenerative anaemia, progressive neurological abnormalities and anterior uveitis. It is supported by laboratory findings of a non-regenerative anaemia and leucocytosis with neutrophilia and lymphopenia, serum hyperproteinaemia (greater than 80 g/litre) with a hyperglobulinaemia (40 g/litre and often 50 g/litre) of mainly γ-globulin, globulin-rich pleural fluid and a positive coronavirus antibody titre. The antibody test is problematic and a significant coronavirus titre without relevant clinical signs may not indicate disease. Similarly, cases con-

firmed by histopathological examination of affected organs
have had low coronavirus titres.

Traumatic pleural effusion

Cats involved in road traffic accidents or with other severe
traumatic injuries may develop various types of effusion.
Haemothorax, chylothorax and pneumothorax can be differentiated by radiology and thoracentesis. Cases of spontaneous
idiopathic chylothorax, pseudochylous effusion and pneumothorax which can have very variable responses to therapy are
also encountered. Haemothorax has been reported in cases of
warfarin poisoning but is often accompanied by spontaneous
haemorrhage at other sites.

Other causes of pleural effusion

Congestive heart failure

This results in accumulation of clear to blood-tinged acellular
transudate, with low to moderate protein, in the thorax. The
causes are discussed later.

Lung lobe torsion

This is a rare cause of pleural effusion in the cat. The
underlying cause of torsion is unclear but after thoracentesis
one single lung lobe is often visibly collapsed and consolidated.
Thoractomy and lobectomy are required to provide definitive
diagnosis and to treat the condition.

Nephrotic syndrome

The severe serum hypoproteinaemia that results from the
proteinuria of glomerulonephritis in the nephrotic syndrome
can induce pleural effusion. However, ascites and subcutaneous oedema over the face, limbs and ventral abdomen are
much more common features. Serum albumin levels will be

dramatically depressed, kidney function may be impaired and there will be gross proteinuria.

THORACIC MASSES

Thoracic masses are often accompanied by effusion but even before thoracentesis there may be an indication that a mass is involved in displacement of thoracic viscera (Fig. 4.8). Elevation of the trachea and deviation of the cardiac silhouette are indications of intrathoracic masses.

Thymic lymphosarcoma

Thymic lymphosarcoma is a common cause of effusion in young cats associated with feline leukaemia virus infection. The majority of cases are less than 2 years old and are commonly from areas of increased feline leukaemia virus exposure, such as breeding colonies or multi-cat households. Although the thymic mass is slow growing, the onset of dyspnoea can be acute. It is accompanied by muffling and displacement of heart sounds, pleural effusion, loss of compliance of the anterior rib cage (poor "rib spring"), compression of the oesophagus (causing regurgitation) and occasionally by peripheral lymphadenopathy. Although pleural effusion commonly obscures detail in lateral radiographs, dorsal dis-

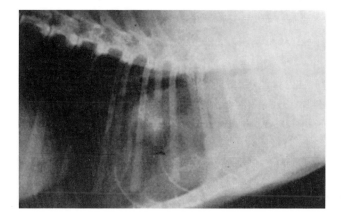

Fig. 4.8
Masses involving the anterior thorax produce effusion with displacement of the trachea dorsally.

placement of the trachea is usually present. Cytology of fluid obtained by thoracentesis usually reveals shed lymphosarcomatous cells and occasionally abnormal peripheral circulating lymphoid cells are also recognized. As over 80% of cats will be feline leukaemia virus positive on ELISA or virus isolation this is a useful diagnostic test.

Diaphragmatic rupture

Diaphragmatic rupture is usually traumatic in origin. There may be signs or history of recent trauma but in some cases signs are delayed. It results in herniation of abdominal viscera into the thoracic cavity (Fig. 4.9), often with pleural effusion. Auscultation and percussion may suggest displacement of thoracic organs and palpation of the abdomen often conveys an impression of emptiness. Radiography followed by paracentesis or oral barium contrast will help in a diagnosis and aid

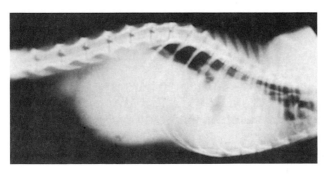

Fig. 4.9
Diaphragmatic rupture can result in herniation of abdominal contents into the thorax.

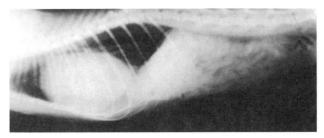

Fig. 4.10 Pericardioperitoneal diaphragmatic hernia is a not uncommon congenital abnormality resulting in herniation of abdominal contents into the pericardium.

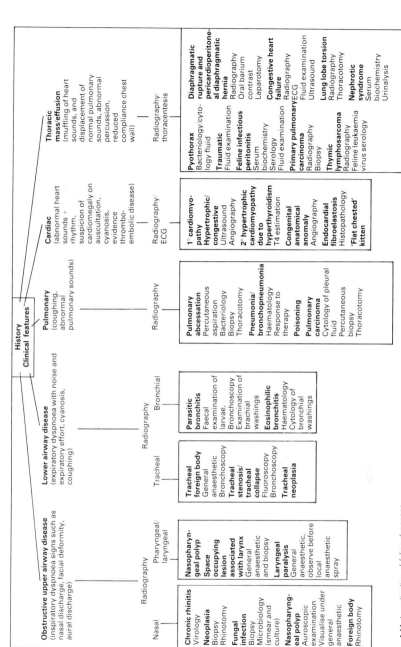

Fig. 4.11 Investigation of feline dyspnoea.

management. In a few cases diaphragmatic tears allow the herniation of only small quantities of tissue such as the liver. Clinical signs of effusion can be slow to develop.

Pericardioperitoneal diaphragmatic hernia

This is an uncommon form of intrathoracic mass and effusion. It is found mainly in young, long-haired cats often with poor growth. There is a congenital connection between the pericardium, diaphragm, and peritoneal cavity. Abdominal contents herniate to surround the heart in a dilated and thickened pericardinal sac (Fig. 4.10). Surgical repair can be successful and the pericardium will return to a normal size.

CARDIAC DISEASE

Congestive heart failure

This is the end result of a range of feline cardiac disorders, and, unlike the dog, ascites and hepatomegaly are not common features. More commonly, cats are presented with dyspnoea resulting from pleural effusion or pulmonary oedema. The most common congenital cardiovascular defects are atrioventricular valve dysplasia, ventricular septal defects, aortic stenosis, patent ductus arteriosus, tetralogy of Fallot and endocardial fibroelastosis. "Fading", stunted growth and signs of cardiac insufficiency are common features in all these conditions.

Cardiomyopathy is relatively common in the cat and tachy-cardia, arrhythmias and thrombo-embolic episodes (e.g. aortic, iliac, renal or cerebral emboli) may be found with or without dyspnoea. The two forms of cardiomyopathy, congestive and hypertrophic can be differentiated by angiography and ultrasound examination. Secondary hypertrophic cardiomy-opathy is also a common sequel to hyperthyroidism caused by a functioning thyroid adenoma. This is a frequent cause of weight loss and wasting in older cats and clinical signs can include profound weight loss, polyphagia, polydipsia, hyperactivity and even jaundice in addition to dyspnoea.

CONCLUSION

A wide variety of conditions cause dyspnoea in the cat (Fig. 4.11). Their differential diagnosis is vital not only for an estimation of prognosis but also for selection of appropriate treatment. Diagnosis can also be very rewarding to the small animal clinician.

ACKNOWLEDGEMENTS

I am grateful to the many colleagues who helped in the preparation of this article, particularly Paul Wotton and Tim Gruffydd-Jones.

CHAPTER 5

Anaemia

RICHARD EVANS AND TIM GRUFFYDD-JONES

INTRODUCTION

Anaemia is a common presenting sign in feline medicine.
More than 10% of cats referred to our clinics have anaemia,
and 7% have profound anaemia, with a haemoglobin concentration on presentation of less than 8.00 g/dl.

Feline anaemia can also be a frustrating clinical problem. A
large proportion of cases remain undiagnosed and the prognosis in those in which a diagnosis is reached is remarkably
poor: more than 80% of cats with anaemia referred to us have
died within 18 months of presentation.

There are a number of reasons why feline anaemia is such
a difficult problem. Cats have a well developed ability to adapt
their lifestyle to compensate for disease processes and therefore
clinical signs may not become apparent until the anaemia is
profound. In addition, poor exercise tolerance is one of the
most important early presenting signs in anaemia in other
species, but this is rarely noticed by cat owners.

Anaemia is a serious problem also because of the nature of
the underlying disease processes with which it is commonly
associated in cats, such as feline leukaemia virus infection
and neoplasms.

Anaemia in the cat, as in any other species, is not a

diagnosis. Rather, anaemia is a clinical sign associated with a number of conditions and if the prognosis is to be assessed correctly and the appropriate treatment is to be instituted it is vital that the animal receives a thorough clinical and laboratory investigation.

DEFINITION OF ANAEMIA

Anaemia is present when a cat's blood haemoglobin concentration is below the lower limit of the normal range (10–15.5 g/dl). Haemoglobin concentration has many advantages as the variable by which anaemia is defined; it is the blood parameter least susceptible to alteration during storage or transit of samples and reliable results can be obtained readily in the practice laboratory.

It is likely that significant differences exist in haemoglobin concentration between breeds of cat and also between individuals within a breed but these have not been investigated and thus rather wide reference values for haemoglobin concentration are accepted. Undoubtedly anaemia will be missed in some individuals that have a high normal haemoglobin concentration so if it is suspected it is particularly valuable to compare new data with any previous determination of haemoglobin concentration.

CLINICAL SIGNS OF ANAEMIA

Signs associated with anaemia can be divided into two categories, those related directly to the presence of anaemia and those caused by underlying disease processes.

SIGNS RELATED TO THE ANAEMIA ITSELF

Pallor of the mucous membranes

This is one of the cardinal indicators of the presence of anaemia, although it may result from cardiovascular dysfunction such as may occur in shock. It is therefore essential to confirm the presence of anaemia by measurement of the packed cell volume or, preferably, the haemoglobin concentration. Particular care is required in the cat also because the appearance of the mucous membranes can be very misleading.

Lethargy and anorexia

These are the most common presenting signs but their nonspecific nature render them of little diagnostic value.

Tachypnoea

Tachypnoea or dyspnoea are rarely presented at rest except in very severe or rapidly developing anaemias or where there has been intrapleural or pulmonary haemorrhage, but may be readily induced by exertion in some cases.

Heat-seeking

Many anaemic cats show increased cold sensitivity or an increased tendency to seek sources of heat.

Pica

Pica, in the form of licking at concrete paths, consuming cat litter, etc. may be encountered and should alert the clinician to the possibility of anaemia. Occasionally severe pica may in itself lead to secondary problems, such as impaction of the intestines in the anaemic cat which develops a craving for cat litter.

Cardiovascular signs

Compensatory reflexes lead to an increase in heart rate and stroke volume and a drop in peripheral resistance so that the heart enters a high output state with an extremely rapid and bounding pulse. The increased cardiac output coupled with the alteration in blood viscosity may give rise to increased turbulence and thus to a haemic murmur.

Pyrexia

Fever is commonly associated with anaemia in cats and may result either from haemolysis or from accompanying diseases.

Hepatomegaly

Enlargement of the liver may be palpable in cats with profound anaemia, irrespective of the cause, and this results from hypoxic damage. In some cats abdominal palpation will elicit pain.

SIGNS RELATED TO UNDERLYING DISEASE

Some clinical signs may be present which provide clues to the type of anaemia involved. Excessive breakdown of red blood cells may lead to splenomegaly. Although a prehepatic jaundice may result from haemolysis, the capacity of the liver to conjugate bilirubin is seldom exceeded.

Examination of the mucous membranes may also reveal muddy discoloration indicative of methaemoglobinaemia or Heinz body anaemia, and petechial haemorrhages suggesting thrombocytopenia. Anaemic cats should be carefully checked for any other evidence of blood loss and it is important to appreciate that haematuria and melaena may be overlooked by owners.

In cats infected with feline leukaemia virus, evidence of neoplasia or of some other leukaemia virus-related non-neoplastic disease such as uveitis or complications of immuno-suppression may be found.

CAUSES OF FELINE ANAEMIA

Anaemia may arise in five ways:

(1) Red cell loss: haemorrhagic anaemia
(2) Abnormal destruction of red blood cells: haemolytic anaemia
(3) Disorganized production of red cells by the bone marrow: dyserythropoiesis
(4) Underproduction of red cells by the bone marrow: hypoplastic or aplastic anaemia depending upon whether the production failure is partial or total
(5) Anaemia associated with systemic disorders

Haemorrhagic and haemolytic anaemias are associated with a marrow erythropoietic response and commonly are referred to as regenerative anaemias. In hypoplastic or aplastic anaemias there is no or minimal evidence of marrow response. Dyserythropoietic anaemias may present some difficulty in classification and diagnosis. When evidence of regeneration is present it will clearly be abnormal in nature (see below). Anaemias secondary to other diseases can be of any of the four types.

HAEMORRHAGIC ANAEMIA

Acute haemorrhage

Acute haemorrhagic anaemia is relatively rare in the cat. Most frequently it is caused by trauma in which case the haemorrhage and its origin will generally be obvious. It is important to remember that it may be some 12 h after bleeding commences before fluid shifts restore the circulating blood volume and that during this period measurements of red cell parameters give no indication of the severity of blood loss.

It may be a further 2–3 days before the erythropoietic response is detectable and until this point the anaemia is normochromic and normocytic. Once the bone marrow erythropoietic response is established the mean corpuscular volume is increased, there is polychromasia, anisocytosis and reticulocytosis, and nucleated red blood cells may be present in the peripheral circulation.

Increased numbers of Howell–Jolly bodies may be present. These are unexpelled nuclear remnants and indicate regeneration or splenic dysfunction. The red cell regeneration is usually accompanied by a similar reaction in the granulocytes expressed as a neutrophilia with left shift.

Congenital and acquired bleeding disorders involving the clotting cascade or the blood platelets occur rarely in the cat and their diagnosis is beyond the scope of this review. However, if the animal has an acquired coagulopathy, warfarin poisoning must be considered. A presumptive diagnosis may be made if there is evidence of warfarin consumption, and if there is a prolonged one-stage prothrombin time. A response to therapy with vitamin K_1 confirms the diagnosis.

Chronic blood loss

Chronic blood loss may occur as the result of persistently bleeding lesions, usually in the urinary or gastrointestinal tracts. In the early stages of chronic blood loss the anaemia is normochromic and macrocytic or normocytic but subsequently may become hypochromic and microcytic if the bleeding is sufficiently prolonged for iron stores to become depleted.

If iron depletion becomes severe marrow aplasia may develop. Iron deficiency anaemia in adult cats rarely results from dietary deficiency but may occur following chronic haemorrhage. Ecto- or endoparasite burdens are unlikely to be sufficiently heavy to produce anaemia apart from occasional exceptionally heavy flea burdens or coccidiosis in kittens.

HAEMOLYTIC ANAEMIA

Anaemia due to excessive red cell destruction is encountered commonly in the cat. Some cases are caused by feline leukaemia virus or parasitism of the red cells by *Haemobartonella felis* but in many the aetiology is uncertain. Anaemia caused by oxidative intoxicants is occasionally encountered.

In most cases it is unlikely that haemolysis will be suspected as the cause of anaemia on the basis of clinical signs.

However, if haemolysis is intravascular and extremely rapid, haemoglobinuria and jaundice may be seen if the capacity of the liver to conjugate bilirubin is exceeded. In these cases the bilirubin will be primarily of the indirect acting unconjugated form. There may also be splenomegaly related to increased breakdown of red blood cells, or extramedullary haematopoiesis and peripheral lymphadenopathy. Occasionally in cases of oxidant poisoning the mucous membranes appear muddy.

Once well established all these anaemias are characterized by evidence of a marrow response. There is a marked reticulocytosis which is indicated by the presence of anisocytosis, polychromasia and an increased mean cell volume. Late normoblasts (nucleated red blood cells) may appear in the circulation and Howell–Jolly bodies may be present in large numbers (Figs 5.1–5.4).

Evidence of a generalized bone marrow response may also be present in the form of neutrophilia, often with a left shift, and thrombocytosis. It is important to appreciate that a

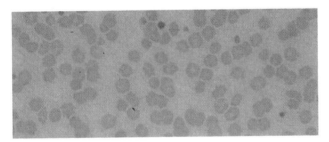

Fig. 5.1 An anaemia with some bone marrow response. Occasional polychromatic cells are present and some cells contain Howell–Jolly bodies. This animal was also iron-deficient and there is moderate hypochromasia: note the prominent area of central pallor in many of the cells.

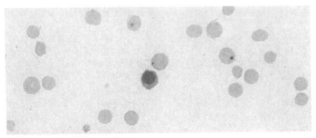

Fig. 5.2 An anaemia with a strong regenerative response. A nucleated red blood cell is present in addition to Howell–Jolly bodies, anisocytosis and polychromasia.

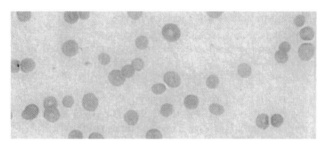

Fig. 5.3 An anaemia with a marrow response showing anisocytosis and marked polychromasia of the majority of cells.

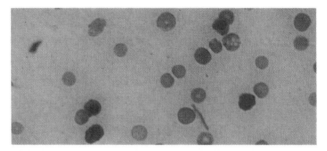

Fig. 5.4 Anaemia with a large number of nucleated red blood cells associated with myelophthisis.

leucocytosis or left shift in such cases is not necessarily indicative of infection.

The bone marrow response takes some 2–3 days to become established so that animals with acute haemolysis may present before there is any haemotological evidence of regeneration.

Feline infectious anaemia

Feline infectious anaemia refers to the haemolytic anaemia associated with parasitism of the red cells by *Haemobartonella felis*.

The most suitable stain for identifying the organisms in the practice laboratory is Giemsa but meticulous care during the staining procedure is essential to avoid artefacts. Top quality rapidly air-dried, unfixed smears are required and these should be prepared as soon after collection of the blood sample as possible. The slide is stained in an inverted position so that any deposits fall to the bottom of the droplet. Smears are stained for 2 h and the slide is examined under oil immersion.

The parasites appear as faintly to strongly reddish-purple ring-like or coccoid structures on the surface of the cell and as dots or rods around the periphery of the cell (Fig. 5.5). Occasionally they may lie free in the intercellular space because of degeneration of cells or detachment of the organism from the cells.

Red cell destruction in feline infectious anaemia appears to be primarily extravascular, with sequestration of red cells in spleen, liver and lung with erythrophagocytosis occurring in the spleen. It also appears that splenic macrophages can remove the parasite from the surface of the red cells, a feature which may account for the rapid increase in packed cell volume which is sometimes seen as the parasitaemia is cleared. Some intravascular destruction of red blood cells may occur since cases may show reduced plasma haptoglobin levels.

The severity of clinical signs associated with *H. felis* infection is very variable. Clinically inapparent infection can occur and in some surveys of normal, non-anaemic cats the organism has been found in a significant proportion of individuals. In some cases an acute clinical presentation is seen but in others the disease runs a more chronic undulant course with repetitive cycles of haemolysis and progressive decline in haemoglobin levels.

The acute disease presents with a haemolytic crisis. The animal is depressed, anorexic, weak and often collapsed; it may show marked tachypnoea. Jaundice and haemoglobinuria

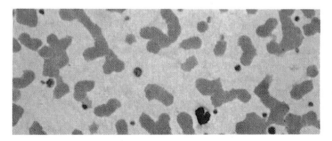

Fig. 5.5 Haemolytic anaemia. This film shows many *Haemobartonella felis* on the surface of the red blood cells. Occasional Howell–Jolly bodies are also present. Autoagglutination of the red cells is also prominent. Although classically associated with immune-mediated anaemias autoagglutination may be encountered in other feline anaemias and is quite commonly seen with *H. felix* infection.

may be noted but are often absent even in the acute form of the condition. Animals may die very soon after signs appear but a significant proportion of animals do survive an acute haemolytic crisis.

Diagnosis depends upon the demonstration of the presence of an anaemia with a marrow response and of the presence of the parasite. Since the peak of the parasitaemia precedes the haemolytic episode and the parasite disappears rapidly from the blood during haemolysis, demonstration of the organism may prove very difficult. At least five blood films should be examined over a period of 5–10 days before negative findings are accepted. Animals with feline infectious anaemia are often infected with feline leukaemia virus and it is therefore wise to determine the patient's virus status.

Most cats affected with feline infectious anaemia become carriers. In experimental studies attempts to induce relapses by putting carriers under stress have proved unsuccessful and apparent relapses probably reflect failure to treat the initial infection adequately allowing persistence of the organism. It is therefore important that treatment should be continued for several weeks.

The epidemiology of feline infectious anaemia is poorly understood. Occasionally, small epizootics occur in colonies but it is usually a sporadic disease of individual cats. The mode of transmission is not known although congenital infection has been demonstrated. Ectoparasite infestation and cat bites have also been suggested but it seems likely that other modes of transmission are involved. Infected animals develop antibodies to the parasite but it is not known whether these protect against reinfection or indeed whether they may contribute to clearance of the parasite from the blood or to red cell destruction.

The treatment of feline infectious anaemia has two components:

(1) Every effort should be made to eliminate the causal organism. The drug of choice is oxytetracycline at a dosage of 20 mg/kg bodyweight three times daily. Initially this should be administered intravenously, followed by oral therapy for at least 14 days. Examinations for the presence of the parasite in the blood should be made before discontinuing the therapy and again some days after cessation.

(2)   Supportive measures such as blood transfusion may be vital to the survival of the animal. The administration of haematinics is not indicated. The provision of vitamins and high protein diet may be of value.

The majority of our cases of feline infectious anaemia have also been positive for feline leukaemia virus and have died shortly after presentation but the prognosis for the first opinion cases may be better.

Feline leukaemia virus

Cats infected with feline leukaemia virus may show regenerative anaemia, presumed to be of haemolytic origin, in the absence of evidence of *Haemobartonella* species or any other feline leukaemia-related disease. The mechanism of this haemolysis is not clear although damage to the cell membrane by virus budding and antibody-mediated destruction of cells expressing viral antigen are possibilities. The anaemia may be transient and may pass unnoticed. Affected cats may undergo recurrent haemolytic episodes but eventually marrow failure may develop.

Although the prognosis in the long term is poor, affected cats may remain relatively free of clinical signs apart from occasional bouts of transient, mild anaemia for a considerable time. Corticosteroids appear to have a beneficial effect in some cases, possibly through suppression of immune-mediated destruction of red cells.

Heinz body haemolytic anaemia

Cats are very susceptible to oxidative insults to haemoglobin which produce methaemoglobinaemia with Heinz body formation and intravascular haemolysis. Heinz bodies appear as large, usually single, refractile non-staining bodies on Leishman stained smears. They can be readily demonstrated by the use of supravital stains (Fig. 5.6).

A significant proportion (up to 10%) of red blood cells in normal cats may contain these bodies. They are thought to consist of denatured haemoglobin. A number of toxins have

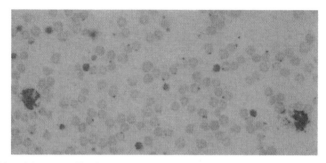

Fig. 5.6 Haemolytic anaemia. This film, stained supravitally with brilliant cresyl blue, shows abundant discrete, blue, peripherally placed Heinz bodies. This cat had been given paracetamol by the owner and methaemoglobinaemia was marked, the blood being chocolate-brown.

been implicated as causes of Heinz body anaemias, most commonly methylene blue or paracetamol. Fortunately urinary antiseptics containing methylene blue are no longer in common use and this is now rarely, if ever, encountered. Administration of paracetamol to cats by misguided owners is not uncommon. Facial oedema is also a feature of the intoxication.

Cats given methylene blue which survive the acute insult develop a marrow response. The drug should be withdrawn and supportive therapy instituted. In the case of paracetamol a single tablet is often sufficient to cause death within hours.

We have encountered a number of cases of Heinz body anaemia in cats with gastrointestinal stasis or obstruction and it would appear that in this situation absorption of intestinal products can lead to autointoxication. This has also been reported as a feature of the Key–Gaskell syndrome (dysautonomia), presumably caused by the associated gut stasis, but is unusual in the authors' experience.

Other rare haemolytic anaemias

Congenital erythropoietic porphyria, which is an hereditary disorder of haem biosynthesis, has been reported in the cat. This causes anaemia with extravascular haemolysis and with pinkish brown staining of teeth and bones caused by the accumulation of porphyrins. Affected animals may show photosensitization, the urine is dark and fluoresces under ultraviolet light. A spontaneous Heinz body anaemia of unknown mechanism has been reported in Siamese kittens.

Haemolytic anaemia of uncertain cause: immune-mediated anaemia

Many cases of haemolytic anaemia in the cat have no identifiable cause. In view of the difficulty of making a definitive diagnosis it it thought that some of these may be associated with *H. felis* infection but others may be immune-mediated.There are a number of reports claiming to demonstrate autoimmune haemolytic anaemia in the cat but we believe that the status of autoimmune anaemia in the cat remains uncertain, although it seems highly likely that such anaemias occur.

There are considerable problems involved in making a diagnosis of autoimmune anaemia in the cat. First, spherocytosis is impossible to detect because of the extremely globular shape of the normal feline erthrocyte. Secondly, not only is the demonstration of anti-red cell antibodies fraught with difficulty but also the significance of these findings is questionable.

Interpretation of the Coombs tests has been hindered by lack of knowledge of feline red cell antigens, although recently a comprehensive blood grouping system in cats has been described by Auer and Bell (1980). Positive Coombs test results may be obtained in many animals infected with feline leukaemia virus or with *H. felis*. It is difficult to know whether these represent false positives due to membrane abnormalities or whether they are genuinely caused by anti-erythrocyte autoantibodies.

Even if these results do reflect the presence of anti-red cell antibodies it is uncertain whether they have any role in the genesis of the anaemia or whether they are incidental findings. A further complication of laboratory assessment is caused by the spontaneous autoagglutination of red blood cells which appears to occur in many anaemic cats irrespective of the cause of the anaemia and which precludes some tests for autoimmune disease.

In the authors' experience many of the cats in which a tentative diagnosis of immune-mediated anaemia has been made have subsequently developed a myeloproliferative disorder or have been shown to be feline leukaemia virus-positive, which reinforces doubts about the validity of tests currently available.

There are reports of the occurrence of the polysystemic autoimmune disease systemic lupus erythematosus in the cat and in other species immune-mediated anaemia may be a feature of the syndrome. Glomerulonephritis, bullous skin disease, polyarthritis with shifting lameness, leucopenia and throbocytopenia may also be present. Again the authors consider that the validity of tests to detect systemic lupus erythematosus in cats has not been established.

If investigation reveals an anaemia with a marrow response and feline infectious anaemia, haemorrhage and the toxic causes of haemolysis have all been eliminated, then administration of prednisolone may be indicated. High initial doses, of 2–4 mg/kg bodyweight daily in divided doses, are required, which are gradually reduced over 8 weeks to alternate day therapy with 0.125 mg/kg. Although a high proportion of patients may show a short term response to this regime the long term prognosis in these cases remains poor.

DYSERYTHROPOIETIC ANAEMIAS

Iron deficiency anaemia: hypochromic anaemia

Iron deficiency anaemia is uncommon in the cat. It may be a late feature of the anaemia of chronic haemorrhage or it may occur in sucking kittens just before weaning. Iron levels in the milk of the cat are only marginally adequate and iron deficiency anaemia is therefore encountered from time to time. The anaemia is usually normocytic and normochromic although occasionally mild hypochromasia is encountered.

Kittens are born with a packed cell volume close to that of adults (0.35–0.45 litres/litre) which then declines progressively to a level of 0.20–0.25 litres/litre at around 4–6 weeks of age before increasing gradually to reach adult levels again by 6 months of age. The deficiency is rarely sufficiently severe to present as a clinical problem but occasionally litters or, more commonly, a few individuals in a litter, may have lower levels and fail to thrive. Treatment is then required and iron supplements should be given.

Myelophthisis

A variety of marrow disorders characterized by abnormal cell development and maturation occur in cats. Many of these cases are associated with feline leukaemia virus infection. In any neoplastic condition in which there is infiltration and replacement of the bone marrow by neoplastic cells, myelophthisic anaemia may be encountered. The neoplastic process may involve lymphoid leukaemia, any of the granulocyte precursors, megakaryocyte precursors or undifferentiated stem cells. The anaemia is characterized by the presence of nucleated red cells in the peripheral blood in the absence of a significant reticulocytosis (Fig. 5.7).

Signs indicative of anaemia may first prompt blood examination which reveals the presence of abnormal circulating cells. Affected cats may also show more vague signs of intermittent pyrexia, inappetance, progressive weight loss and vomiting. The diagnosis is confirmed by examination of marrow biopsies.

Myelophthisic anaemia may also occur in feline leukaemia virus-infected cats due to myelofibrosis or myelosclerosis in which there is replacement of the medullary cavity by fibrous or sclerotic tissue. In severe cases the thickening of the cortical bone may be evident radiographically. Treatment of these cases is unlikely to be feasible and they have a poor prognosis.

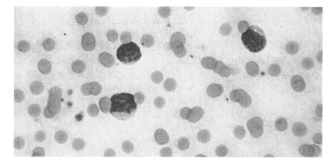

Fig. 5.7 Neoplastic lymphoid cells present in the peripheral blood of a cat with anaemia secondary to lymphoid leukaemia.

Lead poisoning

Lead poisoning in cats is uncommon but is encountered from time to time. It presents as a normochromic normocytic or macrocytic mildly hypochromic anaemia which may be accompanied by gastrointestinal or nervous signs. Examination of a blood film in many cases reveals the presence of large numbers of nucleated red blood cells. Basophilic stippling of red cells may also be present, together with increased numbers of Heinz bodies. Basophilic stippling is not pathognomonic of lead poisoning nor is it invariably present in the condition and it may occur in any strongly regenerative anaemia.

Lead poisoning should be seriously considered when more than 40/1000 red cells show stippling. Anticoagulation of the blood with EDTA greatly reduces the amount of basophilic stippling seen and smears for examination for stippling are best made immediately and without any anticoagulant. Both blood and urine lead levels are then increased. It is believed the blood lead levels reflect absorption while urinary lead levels are more appropriate for the monitoring of treatment.

Microcytic hypochromic anaemia

As mentioned above, any prolonged regenerative anaemia may eventually lead to marrow exhaustion and development of a microcytic, hypochromic picture. This is particularly likely to occur in the case of haemorrhagic anaemias in which red blood cells are lost from the body.

ANAEMIA ASSOCIATED WITH MARROW HYPOPLASIA OR APLASIA

Marrow failure is a common cause of anaemia in the cat. In a moderate proportion of these cases the aetiology is apparent; feline leukaemia virus infection, intoxication (for example, with chloramphenicol or aromatic hydrocarbons), chronic inflammatory disease or chronic renal failure may underlie the depression of erythropoiesis. Bone marrow exhaustion may also lead to aplasia as a terminal feature of regenerative anaemias. In many cases however the aetiology remains obscure.

Depression of bone marrow activity most commonly affects all the haemopoietic cell series. Thus generally there is a pancytopenia and it is this situation which is described as aplastic or hypoplastic anaemia. Since this pancytopenia is in fact secondary to the primary marrow condition the correct description is in fact marrow hypoplasia or aplasia. Since both white cells and blood platelets have substantially shorter life spans than do the red cells affected animals may present with recurrent or overwhelming infections or with purpura before the anaemia is well developed. The anaemia is normochromic and normocytic and reticulocytes (and therefore polychromatic red cells) are absent or present only in very low numbers depending upon whether there is marrow hypoplasia or total aplasia. A number of possible causes of hypoplastic or aplastic anaemia are recognized. One of the most commonly diagnosed is feline leukaemia virus.

Absence of polychromatic cells (reticulocytes) and normoblasts in blood smears indicates non-regeneration by the marrow but one recent report suggests that in at least a proportion of these cases there may be macrocytosis, suggesting that the anaemia should be more correctly termed dyserythropoietic. Although there may be a temporary improvement following blood transfusion the prognosis for these cases is extremely poor.

Feline marrow appears to be particularly sensitive to depression by toxic factors. The possible development of marrow failure following chloramphenicol therapy is well recognized. This is a dose-related phenomenon and prolonged treatment is necessary to result in toxicity in most individuals. However, idiosyncratic reactions may occur in some individuals following shorter courses of chloramphenicol and possibly after many other drugs. In view of this potential problem chloramphenicol is contraindicated in cats with anaemia. Oestrogens may also depress the bone marrow in cats and there may be other unrecognized toxins which have a similar effect.

Bone marrow biopsy will confirm the diagnosis. The marrow may be replaced by fat often giving a dry tap but when marrow is obtained it will be hypocellular with reduction in the activity of all cell series. In a small proportion of cases only erythropoiesis will be affected. The condition is then known as pure red cell aplasia and this presents with a normochromic normocytic anaemia with reduced reticulocyte numbers but the white cell and platelet populations remain normal.

ANAEMIA SECONDARY TO SYSTEMIC DISEASES

The anaemias associated with systemic diseases may arise as a result of any of the mechanisms already discussed or by a combination of them. Often they present a wide variety of haematological features and may defy clear cut classification. The major reason for discussing them together is to emphasize the importance of searching thoroughly for evidence of under-lying disease before attempting to interpret the haematological findings. It is the signs of the underlying disorder which are usually the key to reaching the diagnosis in these cases. The animal may be presented because of the anaemia, or it may be an incidental finding on clinical or laboratory examination.

Chronic renal disease

Hypoplastic anaemia of a mild degree is a common feature in cats with chronic renal failure, although it may be masked by dehydration. It is caused by a combination of reduced production of erythropoietin and toxic depression of the marrow by the waste products of protein metabolism together with decreased red cell life span. Haematinics and anabolic steroids are ineffective in treatment which should be directed to the management of the renal condition.

Anaemia associated with neoplasia

Approximately half of all cats with lymphosarcoma show a non-regenerative anaemia. A similar type of anaemia may also be seen associated with other types of neoplasia.

Anaemia associated with chronic inflammatory disease

A mild to moderate hypoplastic anaemia is often a feature of chronic inflammatory diseases but this rarely contributes significantly to the clinical presentation. Such an anaemia is encountered in feline infectious peritonitis and many septic processes. Reduced red cell life span and direct depression of erythroid precursors are important factors in the development of the anaemias. In some bacterial infections iron is used as a substrate and this may deplete body iron stores. In addition iron may be sequestered by the animal and this further contributes to the anaemia. Haematinics containing iron are contraindicated in these cases.

Microangiopathic anaemia

Mechanically induced haemolysis may occur because of direct red cell damage in cavernous tumours, notably haemangiosarcomas or as a result of shredding of red cells by fibrin networks in disseminated intravascular coagulation. In both cases schistocytes (red cell fragments) and poikilocytes are present. In disseminated intravascular coagulation the whole blood clotting time, the one stage prothrombin time and the kaolin cephalin clotting time are all prolonged. Clot retraction is poor and the platelet count is reduced. Fibrinogen is depleted and fibrin degradation products are present.

INVESTIGATION OF THE ANAEMIC CAT

It is clear that speculative treatment of cats on the basis of a clinical suspicion of anaemia is not jusified. It is essential to establish not only that anaemia is present but also what type and to determine the underlying cause before any assessment can be made of the most appropriate treatment and the likely outcome (Fig. 5.8). Indeed, speculative treatment, particularly with haematinics, before a diagnosis has been reached, is contraindicated since the consequent changes in haematological features may subsequently render accurate diagnosis impossible. Furthermore haematinics are specifically contraindicated in some cases of anaemia – such as in anaemia associated with septic infections.

Every anaemic cat should be thoroughly investigated on first presentation. A full medical history is required and this should be followed by a thorough clinical examination with particular attention paid to the presence of signs relating to the underlying disease conditions which have been discussed above. If there is clinical suspicion of the presence of anaemia this should be confirmed by determination of haemoglobin concentration or packed cell volume which should be inter- preted in the light of a concomitant plasma protein determi- nation. The presence of mild or moderate anaemia, and the severity of any anaemia, can only be established by the measurement of one of these values.

If an anaemia is discovered the authors suggest the following minimum tests:

(1)   Packed cell volume, haemoglobin and red blood cell counts
(2)   White blood cell count with differential and assessment of platelet numbers
(3)   Examination of blood smears for assessment of red blood cell morphology
(4)   A feline leukaemia virus test
(5)   Further tests depending on the characterization of the anaemia assessed from (1) and (3).

A red blood cell count is required for determination of the red cell indices, indicating whether the mean cell volume is normal, increased or decreased and whether there is hypochromasia. Examination of the blood film is essential and will provide further evidence of whether the red cells are normochromic or hypochromic and whether there are any features of a marrow response of dyshaematopoiesis. The presence and nature of any red cell inclusions or of H. felis may be noted as may abnormalities of red cell morphology. If the presence of Heinz bodies is suspected, a suspicion which may be increased by muddy brown cyanosis of the patient or chocolate brown discoloration of the blood sample, examination of a smear stained supravitally with new methyl- ene blue or brilliant cresyl violet is useful.

The physiology of cat reticulocytes is somewhat unusual in

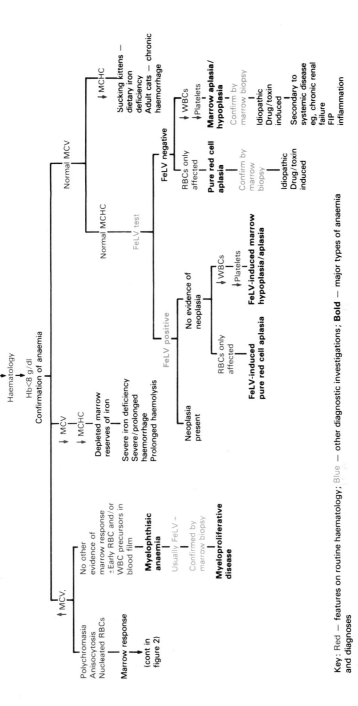

Clinical suspicion of anaemia
↓
Haematology
↓
Hb<8 g/dl
↓
Confirmation of anaemia

↓MCV.
↓
Polychromasia
Anisocytosis
Nucleated RBCs
↓
Marrow response
↓
(cont in figure 2)

No other evidence of marrow response
±Early RBC and/or WBC precursors in blood film
↓
Myelophthisic anaemia
Usually FeLV −
Confirmed by marrow biopsy
↓
Myeloproliferative disease

↓MCV
↓MCHC
↓
Depleted marrow reserves of iron
Severe iron deficiency
Severe/prolonged haemorrhage
Prolonged haemolysis

Normal MCV

Normal MCHC
↓
FeLV test

FeLV positive
↓
Neoplasia present
↓
No evidence of neoplasia
↓
RBCs only affected
↓
FeLV-induced pure red cell aplasia
↓
↓WBCs
↓Platelets
↓
FeLV-induced marrow hypoplasia/aplasia

FeLV negative
↓
RBCs only affected
↓
Pure red cell aplasia
Confirm by marrow biopsy
↓
Idiopathic
Drug/toxin induced
↓
↓WBCs
↓Platelets
↓
Marrow aplasia/ hypoplasia
Confirm by marrow biopsy
↓
Idiopathic
Drug/toxin induced
Secondary to systemic disease eg, chronic renal failure
FIP
inflammation

↓MCHC
↓
Sucking kittens — dietary iron deficiency
Adult cats — chronic haemorrhage

Key: Red — features on routine haematology; Blue — other diagnostic investigations; **Bold** — major types of anaemia and diagnoses

Fig. 5.8 Protocol for investigating anaemia in cats: 1. *(see also Fig. 5.12)*.

that they have a rather long maturation time in the peripheral circulation and new and old reticulocytes appear morphologically different. Only young, coarsely reticulate cells correspond to polychromatic red cells. Thus reticulocyte counts are difficult to perform and to interpret. A count of polychromatic red cells is therefore a better index of recent erythropoietic activity.

Establishment of the feline leukaemia virus status is very helpful in all anaemic cats. It is important to do this early in the laboratory investigation since feline leukaemia is the single most important cause of anaemia in cats and decisions about the desirability of treatment or of euthanasia will often be made on the basis of this result. It must however be remembered when considering euthanasia that a proportion of anaemic leukaemia virus-positive cats, particularly those with haemolytic disease, may have a reasonable prognosis at least in the short term.

If the mean corpuscular volume is increased or there is evidence of a marrow response in the form of anisocytosis, polychromasia, reticulocytosis and possibly normoblasts the following possibilities must be considered:

(1) *Haemorrhagic anaemia*. The cat should be carefully checked for evidence of blood loss. If substantial haemorrhage has occurred a reduced plasma protein concentration may be found. The cause of the haemorrhage should then be investigated.

(2) *Haemolysis*. The presence of poikilocytes, schistocytes, Heinz bodies or autoagglutination of red cells on the blood film will support this suspicion. If Heinz bodies are present the possibility of exposure to oxidant intoxicants or of gut stasis must be considered. A fresh blood smear should be examined for *H. felis*. If poikilocytes and schistocytes (Fig. 5.9) are present immune-mediated or mechanical haemolysis should be considered and the presence of autoagglutination supports a suspicion of immunological involvement. If disseminated intravascular coagulation is suspected clinical evidence of haemorrhage, thromboembolic organ failure or an underlying cause will be valuable. Detailed haemostatic evaluation is needed to confirm the presence of disseminated intravascular coagulation.

(3) *Dyserythropoiesis*. A low mean corpuscular haemoglobin concentration with hypochromasia, a high normoblast count

out of proportion to the reticulocyte count and abnormal morphology of the blood cells indicates dyshaematopoiesis.

If the mean corpuscular haemoglobin and mean cell volume are low with hypochromasia evident on examination of the smear the possibility of a dietary deficiency, particularly of iron in young kittens, should be investigated. A long term haemorrhagic or haemolytic anaemia leading to marrow exhaustion should also be considered.

If features of dyshaematopoiesis are present in the absence of any evidence of hypochromic anaemia, particularly if abnormal circulating cells are identified, the morphology of the platelets and white blood cells should be carefully checked and a marrow biopsy should be obtained.

(4) *Marrow failure*. Anaemia in the absence of polychromasia, anisocytosis and changes in the derived red cell indices indicates marrow failure and is the other major indication for marrow biposy (Figs 5.10 and 5.11).

BONE MARROW BIOPSY

General anaesthesia or sedation is necessary for this technique and although this may seem hazardous, the authors have experienced no anaesthetic deaths in over 50 cats from which marrow biopsies have been obtained, despite the presence of profound anaemia in most cases. Strict asepsis must be observed particularly since many of these cats are immunosuppressed.

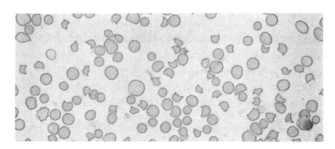

Fig. 5.9 Haemolytic anaemia showing mechanical red cell damage. In this film from a cat with disseminated intravascular coagulation, many mechanically damaged and irregularly shaped red cells (poikilocytes) and angular red cell fragments (schistocytes) are present.

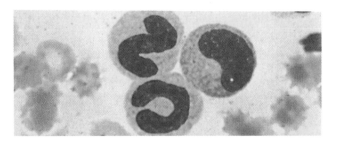

Fig. 5.10 Anaemia secondary to chronic granulocytic leukaemia. The leucocyte content of the peripheral blood is dominated by metamyelocyte, band and mature neutrophils, many of which show abnormal morphology.

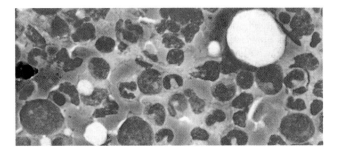

Fig. 5.11 Bone marrow from a severely anaemic cat with chronic granulocytic leukaemia showing marked hypercellularity of the marrow which is dominated by myeloid cells. Erythroid precursors are few in number.

Specially designed paediatric marrow biopsy needles with an internal stilette are essential and these are introduced into the shaft of the femur through the trochanteric fossa or the iliac crest. Marrow is aspirated into a 20 ml syringe containing a small quantity of citrate using sudden application of suction to minimize blood contamination. The marrow is smeared on slides and immediately fixed in methanol. Interpretation of marrow cytology requires specialized experience (Fig. 5.12).

MANAGEMENT OF ANAEMIA

The need to appreciate that anaemia is not a diagnosis in itself has already been mentioned. It is therefore clear that specific treatment of the underlying cause of the anaemia is essential.

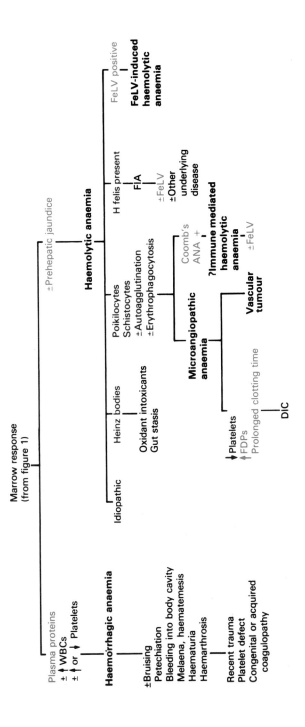

Fig. 5.12 Protocol for investigating anaemia in cats: 2. *(continued from Fig 5.8)*

Key: Red — features on routine haematology; Blue — other diagnostic investigations; **Bold** — major types of anaemia and diagnoses

One situation deserves special consideration: the feline leukaemia virus-positive anaemic cat. If there is a severe hypoplastic or aplastic anaemia or there is a frankly leukaemic blood picture, possibly corroborated by marrow biopsy findings, the prognosis is so poor that in the authors' view euthanasia should be recommended. Even with aggressive supportive therapy including blood transfusions these cats are unlikely to live more than a month or two.

However, the outlook for the feline leukaemia virus-positive cat showing evidence of regeneration is considerably better. In many cases the apparent haemolytic episodes may be transient and although further episodes may occur, a significant proportion of these cases will survive relatively free of clinical signs for some time. Eventually they may develop an aplastic or hypoplastic anaemia or some other leukaemia virus-related disease. Owners of such cats may decide against euthanasia, but the cats are probably lifelong carriers of the virus and it is important to emphasize their infectious nature and the need to prevent transmission to other cats.

A significant proportion of anaemic cats defy definitive diagnosis despite a thorough clinical and haematological investigation. Although the prognosis for such cases is usually poor, empirical supportive therapy is indicated as outlined below. It is important that the clinician should continue to monitor these cats both clinically and by periodic blood examination (at least once every month) since the cause of the anaemia may become apparent in time. Some of the measures outlined below may also be useful as general supportive therapy in addition to the specific treatments for anaemias already mentioned.

SPECIFIC HAEMATINICS

Haematinics should not be administered before a definite diagnosis has been achieved and then only if there is some specific indication. This is very rare in the cat, the major indication being the administration of iron to correct iron deficiency and hypochromasia, usually in kittens. Most commonly iron-dextran is used but since this preparation is painful to administer the authors prefer ferrous sulphate tablets.

Iron administration is not indicated if the mean corpuscular haemoglobin concentration is normal except following haemorrhage when there may be some depletion of marrow iron stores. Furthermore, in some forms of anaemia, most notably those associated with bacterial infection and an inflammatory response in which iron reserves are sequestered, the use of haematinics is contraindicated.

ANABOLIC STEROIDS

Androgenic steroids have a specific stimulant action on erythropoiesis probably via increased erythropoietin levels. They are therefore of some value in marrow aplasia or hypoplasia. A dose at the upper limit of the therapeutic range should be given once weekly for 6 weeks, with regular monitoring of peripheral blood to assess the response. Nandrolone is the agent of choice but unfortunately the response is often poor in cats and such anaemias carry a poor prognosis. In all other anaemias androgens are contraindicated since overstimulation of the marrow can lead to marrow exhaustion.

CORTICOSTEROIDS

In view of the difficulties in confirming a diagnosis of immune-mediated anaemia, corticosteroids may be indicated for cats with haemolytic anaemia for which no definitive diagnosis has been made, particularly if there is circumstantial evidence of autoimmune disease such as schistocytosis or autoagglutination.

An immune-mediated mechanism is thought to be involved in some forms of hypoplastic or aplastic anaemia and these may respond to corticosteroids. Treatment with these drugs may be justified in cases of marrow failure which do not respond to anabolic steroids.

SUPPORTIVE AND SYMPTOMATIC TREATMENT

Supportive therapy in the form of the provision of a balanced palatable diet rich in proteins, minerals and vitamins may

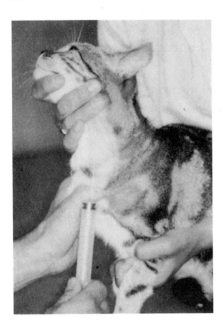

Fig. 5.13
Cat restrained for jugular venepuncture on an examination table. The assistant restrains both front legs with one hand.

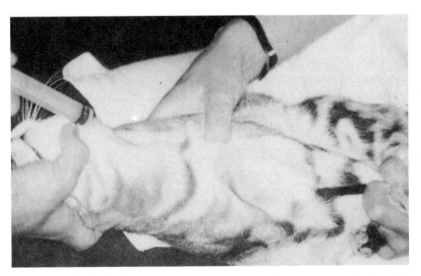

Fig. 5.14 Cat restrained in dorsal recumbency for jugular venepuncture. The cat is placed on the knee of the assistant who sits on a chair. All four legs are held by the assistant's left hand while the right hand is used to raise the jugular vein. The method is preferred by many individuals who bleed cats regularly. It is very well tolerated by most cats and can be used to obtain large volumes of blood for transfusion.

be helpful, but the most important treatment is a blood transfusion.

Blood transfusion

The main indication for blood transfusion is as a supportive measure while the underlying cause of the anaemia is receiving specific treatment, such as in cats infected with *H. felis*. Another indication is for cats with hypoplastic or aplastic anaemia of indeterminate cause while empirical treatment with marrow stimulants is begun or attempts are made to make a specific diagnosis.

Transfusions may also be required for cats which are first presented with life-threatening anaemia requiring immediate treatment although this is relatively uncommon in view of the cat's ability to compensate for anaemia. In such cases transfusion may change the blood picture, thus masking the underlying cause.

Feline blood cannot be stored satisfactorily and must be administered as soon after collection as possible. Thirty to fifty millilitres of blood are collected from a feline leukaemia virus-tested donor by jugular venepuncture (Figs 5.13–5.15)

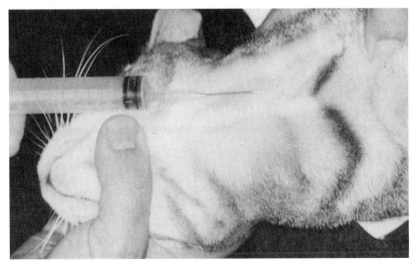

Fig. 5.15 Close-up shows the position of the jugular furrow.

into one ninth by volume of acid-citrate-dextrose (which can be obtained from a blood transfusion collection bag). Cross matching is impractical and in view of the need to transfuse the blood with the minimum delay and the rarity of a reaction following the first transfusion, a test dose is not used. Transfusions may be repeated but not more than 3 days later without risk of a transfusion reaction.

REFERENCES AND FURTHER READING

Alsaker, R. D., Laber, J., Stevens, J. & Perman, V. (1977). *Journal of the American Veterinary Medical Association* **170**, 39.

Auer, L. & Bell, K. (1980). *Animal Blood Groups Biochemistry and Genetics* **11**, 63.

Cotter, S. M. (1979). *Journal of the American Veterinary Medical Association* **175**, 1191.

Harvey, J. W. & Gaskin, J. M. (1977). *Journal of the American Animal Hospitals Association* **13**, 28.

Harvey, J. W. & Gaskin, J. M. (1978). *Journal of the American Animal Hospitals Association* **14**, 453.

Mackey, L., Jarrett, W., Jarrett, O. & Laird, H. (1975) *Journal of the National Cancer Institute* **54**, 209.

Onions, D., Jarrett, O., Testa, F., Frassoni, & Toth, S. (1982). *Nature* **296**, 156.

Weiser, M. G. & Kociba, G. J. (1983). *Veterinary Pathology* **20**, 687.

Weiss, D. J. & Krehbiel, J. D. (1983). *American Journal of Veterinary Research* **44**, 1830.

CHAPTER 6

Basics of Feline Nutrition

IVAN BURGER, ANDREW EDNEY
AND DEREK HORROCKS

INTRODUCTION

Until recently, feline medicine has been the poor relation of
veterinary science. Although this situation has improved, the
nutrition of cats has remained rather neglected. It is of
considerable importance to veterinarians who deal regularly
with cats to have a working knowledge and understanding of
their nutritional peculiarities.

NUTRITIONAL CHARACTERISTICS OF THE CAT

Cats and dogs are often grouped together in consideration of
nutrition, feeding and husbandry. As both species are classified zoologically as Carnivora, this approach would seem to
be logical. However, the cat is nutritionally much more a
carnivore than the dog and is dependent upon having at least
some animal-derived tissue in its diet. Nonetheless, over-
nutrition poses the same problems as it does in other
mammalian species and requires as much attention as the
avoidance of dietary deficiencies. Cats are generally more

fussy and selective in their feeding habits than dogs. This can generate more problems, especially with individuals which are ill.

PROTEINS AND AMINO ACIDS

Cats have a higher maintenance protein requirement than many other mammals. The main reason seems to be their profligate rate of amino acid breakdown which increases the need for dietary protein. The cat seems unable to adjust even when receiving a low protein diet.

The amino acid requirements of the cat are broadly similar to those of other species (Burger and Smith, 1990).

Arginine

The effect of arginine deficiency in the cat is particularly unusual and serves to illustrate the uniqueness of this species' nutritional requirements. Rogers and Morris (1979) reported that cats became ill a few hours after eating a single meal of a purified diet which, other than being devoid of arginine, was nutritionally complete. The clinical signs observed included lethargy, hypersalivation, vocalization and ataxia and were caused by hyperammonaemia resulting from a reduction of urea cycle activity.

Arginine is required by the cat to stimulate urea synthesis by providing ornithine which in turn combines with carbamoyl phosphate, the "carrier" of the ammonia resulting from amino acid catabolism. Carbamoyl phosphate and ornithine form citrulline which starts the sequence again (Fig. 6.1). The provision of ornithine or citrulline overcomes the ammonia toxicity, but only citrulline can restore growth rates to normal. The rapidity of the appearance of the signs was far greater than for any other single nutrient omitted from an otherwise balanced diet and even surpassed the effects of water deprivation. The workers commented that only a severe lack of oxygen would have more dramatic effects. Most other mammals also require arginine but they are far less sensitive to a deficiency of this nutrient.

Taurine

Taurine is a simple amino sulphonic acid and the end product of the metabolism of the sulphur amino acids methionine and cystine. It may be involved in many aspects of metabolism but two of the most important are retinal function and bile salt formation. In the former, taurine is thought to act as a neurotransmitter and is possibly necessary in maintaining the structural integrity of the photoreceptor membrane. More recently, taurine has been shown to be necessary for normal reproduction and growth (Sturman *et al.*, 1986) and heart function in cats (Pion *et al.*, 1987).

Cats can synthesize only a limited amount of taurine and must therefore have a dietary supply. A deficiency of dietary taurine eventually results in retinal degeneration and dysfunction, although it is a gradual process and may take many months to produce obvious clinical signs.

The cat is not unique in having a limited capacity for taurine synthesis – low levels have also been reported in other species, including non-human primates and man. However, cats seem

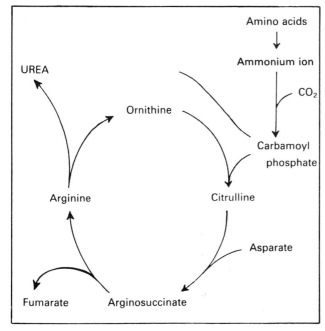

Fig. 6.1
Simplified scheme of the urea cycle.

to compound the problem by using only taurine for bile salt formation and, in contrast to other animals, do not convert to glycine conjugation when the taurine supply is limited. In fact it seems to deplete other tissues, including eventually the retina, to conserve taurine for bile salts. This may explain why the retinal degeneration associated with taurine deficiency has so far been reported only in cats. Taurine is found almost entirely in animal-derived raw materials – little is present in plants.

Cats fed a high proportion of vegetable-derived protein are more likely to fall below the required level but those allowed to catch prey may supplement their diet with animal tissue.

ESSENTIAL FATTY ACIDS

Essential fatty acids are involved particularly in kidney function, reproduction and the structural integrity of the skin. The requirements of most mammals, including the dog, can be satisfied by the provision of linoleic acid in the diet. This is because linoleic acid (a "parent" essential fatty acid) can be converted to more complex "derived" essential fatty acid, such as arachidonic acid, by alternating steps of desaturation and chain elongation.

The cat has only a very limited capacity to carry out one of the desaturation steps and this makes arachidonic acid an essential component of the cat's diet; although it may be required only for the more critical stages of the life cycle, notably reproduction. Linoleic acid is also required and it is likely that an optimal level of linoleic acid decreases the requirement for arachidonic acid. Nevertheless this should not obscure the fact that a diet claimed to be complete and balanced for all cats must contain a certain quantity of arachidonic acid. This means that animal tissues must be included as the derived essential fatty acids, in contrast to linoleic acid, are almost entirely absent from plant materials.

VITAMINS

Vitamin A

The cat is unable to convert carotenes to retinol and thus differs from most other mammalian species (including the dog) which can satisfy at least some of their vitamin A requirement by the conversion of carotenoids to the active compound. The cat must therefore have vitamin A *per se* in its diet and this means a source of animal lipids, as the pre-formed vitamin is not found in plants.

Niacin (nicotinic acid)

Niacin is one of the B complex vitamins and is involved in the formation of a co-factor responsible for oxidation–reduction reactions. The niacin requirement of many mammals can be partly met by the amino acid tryptophan which can be converted to the vitamin, although the degree of conversion varies widely among species. The cat's capacity to convert tryptophan into niacin is negligible. The tryptophan pathway has a branch point where one of the intermediates can go either to niacin synthesis or further breakdown. In the cat the enzyme responsible for the catabolic pathway has a much higher activity than it does in, for example, the rat and therefore diverts tryptophan metabolites from niacin formation to the alternative pathway which can eventually lead to the formation of glucose. There is little practical consequence of this aspect of the normal cat's metabolism as niacin is widely distributed in animal and plant materials, the highest levels being found in animal tissues. It is, however, likely that niacin levels become much more critical when a cat is ill, especially when there are gastrointestinal disturbances.

DIETS FOR CATS

These examples show that the cat is very dependent upon a supply of animal tissue in its food. One theory for this is that the cat has been subjected to little evolutionary pressure to adapt to using plants as a food source because it is a very efficient hunter and in the wild will subsist on what is virtually an "all animal" diet. In this environment a high breakdown of protein may actually represent an advantage in providing the cat with a supply of useable available carbohydrate, which is generally found at only low concentrations in animal tissues. The same reasoning may be applied to the metabolism of tryptophan. It is probable that the cat is not unique in this respect but is merely representative of the strict carnivores. The unusual nutritional profile of the cat results in more stringent dietary requirements than for more omnivorous carnivores such as the dog. It may be possible to design a vegetarian-type diet for cats but it would need very careful supplementation with individual nutrients and would prob- ably still be inadequate for the complete life cycle of the animal. This is mainly because supplementation with pure derived arachidonic acid is not practical unless it is added as a meat-type raw material.

The metabolizable energy (ME) requirements of cats have been reviewed by NRC (1986) and are summarized in Table 6.1. The ME requirements of growing and lactating cats are considerably higher than those of an adult animal, relative to bodyweight. Lactation requirements also vary in relation to litter size.

OVER-NUTRITION

Table 6.1 The metabolizable energy (ME) requirements of cats.

Life stage	Daily ME requirement kcal/kg
Adult – active	80
– inactive	70
Kitten – young	250
– half grown	130
Peak lactation	up to 300
Gestation	100

Obesity

While obesity in the cat is much less common than in the dog, it is still a significant problem in the UK. Critical data are, however, very scarce. Cats in a controlled environment seem well able to control their energy balance and at the Waltham Centre for Pet Nutrition, there is virtually no obesity among a large number of cats fed regularly on an *ad libitum* basis. The situation in domestic cats is even less clear, though one study showed that, among cats attending three small animal veterinary practices, the incidence of obesity ranged from 6.0 to 12.5%. It is said, again without hard evidence, that neutered cats, especially males, show a greater tendency to obesity. What can be said with certainty, however, is that where obesity does occur it is fundamentally a problem of energy balance. A fat, but otherwise healthy, cat eats too much, that is it takes in more energy than it uses, or has done at some time. This state of affairs can only be rectified by reversing the situation, that is by providing less energy in the food than the cat is using. It will, like any other mammal, use its body reserves of fat to make up the deficit and so become slimmer.

Vitamins

While obesity is the most obvious manifestation of over nutrition, there are others which are just as likely to be encountered as cases of under nutrition. The fat-soluble vitamins A, D and E are stored and accumulate in the body so that prolonged exposure to even a moderate excess can cause serious problems. Hypervitaminosis A has been well described, with stiffness and lameness as the main signs resulting from the formation of periarticular exostoses.

Excess vitamin D also results in skeletal abnormalities which will affect the animal's mobility, but here the specific effect is cessation of bone growth and hypertrophic osteodystrophy. Cats fed a high proportion of raw liver in their diet on a regular basis have developed hypervitaminosis A. Regular addition of cod liver oil, sometimes given to such cases, can only supply more fat-soluble vitamins than the cat requires and the well meaning but overzealous use of proprietary vitamin supplements can be equally harmful.

Another condition associated with a surfeit of a normally useful food item is pansteatitis. This generalized inflammation of the body fat has been reported in cats which have been fed a very high level of oily fish such as pilchard. It is thought that high levels of unsaturated fatty acids are the specific cause of the condition through destruction of vitamin E.

Minerals

All minerals should be avoided in excess. Although excess calcium in the diet may not result in much extra calcium being absorbed, it should be carefully avoided. There is evidence that high dietary calcium can impair calcium metabolism and that deficiencies of magnesium and zinc may result from impaired absorption.

Magnesium deficiency causes nervous system disorders, while a shortfall of zinc, which can result from competitive absorption, has serious effects on protein synthesis. This can in turn result in undersize kittens and poor coat condition.

Phosphorus should be considered in conjunction with calcium, and attention paid to the calcium : phosphorus ratio. Thus while an excessive level of phosphorus is in itself undesirable and has been associated with progressive renal disease, all situations where an adverse ratio exists are not necessarily indicative of excess phosphorus in the diet. The classic example is the "all meat" diet with its disastrous Ca : P ratio of 1:15 or 1:20, resulting in severe problems of bone demineralization. Here the correct solution is the supplementation of the diet with sufficient calcium to achieve a Ca : P ratio of about 1:1.

Zinc availability can be a particular problem in dry foods based on vegetable-derived raw materials. Zinc can form insoluble complexes with compounds such as phytic acid, which are found extensively in this type of raw material. Furthermore high levels of calcium and trace elements such as iron and copper in the diet will also reduce the availability of zinc. Skin disease associated with zinc deficiency in dogs fed cereal-based diets has recently been reported (Van den Broeck and Thoday, 1986).

GENERAL PRINCIPLES OF FEEDING ILL CATS

Setting aside conditions which need special dietary adjustment, such as food-induced allergy or lactose intolerance, there are some general feeding principles which can be applied to many illnesses in cats.

Although cats, even when well, have a reputation for being very careful feeders, there are strategies which are often effective when the appetite is depressed by malaise.

It is best to offer cats which are ill small amounts at fairly frequent intervals. (Owners, and occasionally clinic staff, mistakenly keep large amounts of food continuously before an ailing cat). All uneaten food should be removed and disposed of after about 15 min. Fresh supplies can be offered at frequent intervals during the day. Wet food loses its appeal rapidly as it dries out with exposure to room temperatures. Most cats do, however, prefer wet foods, so it is worth adding some water or gravy to the food provided, often depending on the cat's preferences. The re-presenting of food after withholding it will provide new visual cues to the organoleptic system and so help to coax the reluctant feeder.

Cats are sensitive to the temperature of the food they eat. Acceptance usually rises with the temperature of the food, regardless of ambient temperature within normal ranges, up to around 38–39°C (the temperature of any live mammalian prey). Above this the food becomes less attractive to cats. Providing food at blood heat also releases attractive odours which help to encourage a cat to eat. Adding flavours, known to be favoured by particular cats, may help the cat to take a greater interest in food. Owners often mistakenly provide very bland food with very little odour to a cat with a very depressed appetite. What is usually needed, especially for cats with inflammatory conditions of upper respiratory tract, is a food with a penetrating odour, such as sardines or pilchards.

FEEDING ROUTINE

Cats often react unfavourably to influences which disrupt their routine. It is important therefore to feed cats in a location and with utensils they are used to. The cat's usual daily routine should be well established, particularly the time of day when it is normally fed. The main meal of the day should still be provided at this time, although smaller meals on a "little and often" basis can be given after this. However, as cats are basically continuous feeders, they are less of a problem in this respect than dogs.

Although cats are regarded by most people as solitary animals, they often feed enthusiastically in groups or if the food is partly hidden so that it has to be "found". A careful watch has to be maintained to make sure other cats are not preventing free access to the food or that the meal is vomited after feeding.

Nutritional management

Although objective evidence to show that altering a cat's feeding regime improves recovery from particular conditions is scarce, dietary measures are clearly indicated for many disorders. Much of the rationale for this is extrapolated from other species or otherwise applied empirically.

Diabetes mellitus

Treating cats with diabetes mellitus is usually quite rewarding provided that the owners are diligent in their nursing support. Feeding is relatively straightforward as the appetite is usually retained. The objective is to try to stabilize energy intake and output. Prepared foods, especially canned products, have a definite advantage over more haphazard feeding regimes. Canned foods with a high level of palatability and a consistency maintained by careful quality-control methods, are well suited to keeping the energy intake within strict bounds. Semi- or soft-moist foods preserved with humectants such as glycols or simple sugars, must be avoided as they are likely to provoke hyperglycaemic peaks in diabetic individuals.

Contrary to a widely held belief, all carbohydrates are not contraindicated in the diet of diabetics. They can usually accommodate and digest up to 40% of their dietary calories as carbohydrate if they are provided in the form of complex polysaccharides. Thus prepared foods containing potato, rice or wheat are usually quite suitable for feeding to diabetic cats. A recent report on diabetic dogs (Blaxter *et al.*, 1990) suggests that feeding restricted carbohydrate diets to diabetics is an outdated concept. High fibre diets (or dietary supplementation with soluble fibre) may help to improve glycaemic control in this disease.

Individuals which are given insulin by injection need to have their feeding times kept to a strict timetable. An adult cat fed between 70 and 80 kcal/kg over a 24 h period, may still not be able to maintain its bodyweight so adjustments need to be made after careful, frequent assessment. The total calories allowed may be increased by 10% per week until the bodyweight can be maintained. The amount allocated for the day should be divided up so that 25% of the calories are fed each morning and evening and the remainder fed at set intervals throughout the day.

Chronic diarrhoea

Although diarrhoea is but a clinical sign and not a disease in itself, there are some feeding strategies which can be usefully adapted in the management of cats passing frequent fluid faeces. Such cats should be fed small amounts at frequent intervals, avoiding any nutrient known to provoke diarrhoea in the individual concerned. For example, some cats are unable to tolerate liver in their diet. Others are incapable of digesting lactose to any extent. Most adult cats can digest about 3–4 g of lactose daily (lactose-intolerant cats exhaust their lactase supplies long before this). In practical terms this is equivalent to only about 100 ml of ordinary cow's milk. In fact, most prepared foods contain amounts of lactose well within the usual limits, if they contain any at all. It is sensible to withold all milk-based nutrients from the diet of a cat with chronic diarrhoea for a trial period, as in addition to lactose intolerance, a few individuals cannot digest casein, the protein present in milk. This is probably a result of casein acting as an allergen in the gut.

Empirical treatment of feline diarrhoea cases usually includes withholding solid food for a period of 24 h and the restoration of fluid depletion by the administration of electrolyte solutions by mouth or parenterally. In addition to the use of therapeutic agents which absorb fluid from the gut and give some structure to the faeces such as kaolin mixtures and dehydrated potato powder, live yoghurt may be provided for the cat to eat in an effort to colonize the gut with *Lactobacilli* species. Many cats find yoghurts acceptable when mixed with prepared foods or fed on their own.

FOOD ALLERGY

Allergies induced by food are relatively rare in cats. Occasionally allergic reactions to specific problems are seen as skin changes or alimentary disturbances. The most frequent reactions are to casein from milk or its by-products followed by beef or fish protein. The skin and bowel changes are not usually specific enough to differentiate the cause of the allergy or even to establish that they are allergies at all. Food-related allergies can usually be identified by a careful programme of test feeding. Great care has to be taken to make sure only a single protein source such as chicken, fish or rabbit is fed for each test period. Clinical signs should recede when the allergen is withheld (provided there are no secondary complications) and reappear when it is reintroduced. Cats are best hospitalized for this procedure as the discipline of the detective work required is beyond many owners. A period of 5 days exclusive feeding of each putative allergen should be allowed and control of any self-inflicted lesions or secondary infection needs due consideration. Once identified, the allergen must be excluded from the cat's diet for the rest of its life.

FELINE UROLOGICAL SYNDROME

Osborne *et al.* (1984) have made it clear that what is generally known as the feline urological syndrome may well be many different conditions and proper diagnostic criteria must be applied to each case. However, most feline urological syndrome conditions are related to urinary solids coming out of solution. The objective of feeding cats with feline urological syndrome is to create conditions which will reduce the chances of recurrence. These measures are directed towards increasing the water turnover and lowering the cat's urinary pH (Burger, 1987).

Jackson (1970) showed that many cats could be made to increase their water turnover by as much as 70 ml by adding that amount to an already wet diet. If this is combined with the restriction of magnesium in the cat's food, the probability of magnesium ammonium phosphate (struvite) being precipitated is lessened. It is difficult to bring about a significant lowering of urinary pH in cats but the addition of methionine or ammonium chloride to the diet at a level of 0.5–1.0 g/day, will usually make the urine sufficiently acid to retain magnesium compounds in solution. Access to drinking water and with it adequate opportunity for the cat to urinate, is needed at all times to prevent urinary stasis which will only increase the likelihood of urinary solids coming out of solution.

CHRONIC RENAL FAILURE

The difficulties of feeding a protein-restricted regime to cats are greatly magnified when compared with dogs. Low protein diets intended for dogs are not likely to provide sufficient supplies of amino acids and even normal cats are reluctant to eat any diet which supplies less than 20% protein (dry matter).

In order to prevent excess protein being diverted to generate energy, and thus contribute to uraemia in cats with seriously reduced renal function, compromise is usually needed. Wet foods with a protein content of around 30% (dry matter) are normally eaten by those cats which have some appetite remaining. Additional non-protein calories are best provided from fat, preferably of animal origin. Frying food in cooking fat is often an effective way of improving the palatability of the protein-restricted diet. Otherwise non-protein calories may be provided by a supply of fried strips of bacon fat, which most cats find very acceptable.

As with other species, cats with renal failure have a limited ability to excrete phosphorus. As most dietary components are comprised of cellular material, they have a considerable phosphorus content and some supplementation with calcium is necessary. Where the calcium : phosphorus ratio is increased to favour calcium to the extent of about 1.5–2.1, the possibility of secondary hyperparathyroidism can be reduced.

With renal failure, losses via the urine are likely to include water-soluble vitamins. B complex vitamins are needed to offset these losses and to compensate for the poor intestinal absorption and reduced intake associated with a depressed appetite. Little harm is likely to result from the over-provision of vitamins of the B complex, so at least double the cat's normal requirements can be given by mouth. Brewer's yeast or the equivalent can be added to the food provided in amounts of 5 g or more daily.

If a heavy proteinuria is present some additional good quality protein, such as cooked whole egg, added at the rate of 15 g/kg bodyweight daily, will be needed to make good these losses. More protein is always needed when the cat is unable to maintain nitrogen balance. This is indicated where the cat is unable to maintain bodyweight, although it may be eating reasonable amounts of food. Premium grade canned cat food should then be added to the diet provided in increasing amounts while monitoring the individual's blood urea levels.

REFERENCES AND FURTHER READING

Anderson, R. S. (1980). *Nutrition of the Dog and Cat.* Pergamon, Oxford.

Blaxter, A. C., Cripps, P. J. & Gruffyd-Jones, T. J. (1990). *Journal of Small Animal Practice* **31**, 229–233.

Burger, I. H. (1987). *Journal of Small Animal Practice* **28**, 448–452.

Burger, I. H. & Smith, P. M. (1990). Amino acid requirements of adult cats. In *Nutrition, Malnutrition and Dietetics in the Dog and Cat* (eds A. T. B. Edney, H. Meyer & E. Kienzle). Proc. Int. Symp. Hanover Vet. Schl., British Veterinary Association.

Chandler, E. A. & Gaskell, C. J. (eds) (1986). *Feline Medicine*, pp. 339–351. Blackwell, Oxford.

Edney, A. T. B. (ed.) (1987). *Dog and Cat Nutrition.* Pergamon, Oxford.

Gaskell, C. J., Leedale, A. H. & Douglas, S. W. (1975). *Journal of Small Animal Practice* **116**, 117.

Jackson, O. F. (1970). *Journal of Small Animal Practice* **12**, 555.

NRC (1986). *Nutrient Requirements of Cats.* National Research Council, National Academy Press, Washington, DC.

Osborne, C. A., Johnston, G. R., Polzin, D. J., Kruger, J. M., Bell, F. W., Pottenburger, E. M., Feeney, D. A., Stevens, J. B. & McMenomy, M. F. (1984). Feline urologic syndrome, a heterogeneous phenomenon? *Journal of the American Animal Hospital Association.*

Pion, P. D., Kittleson, M. D., Rogers, Q. R. & Morris, J. G. (1987). Myocardial failure in cats associated with low plasma taurine: a reversible cardiomyopathy. *Science* **237**, 764–768.

Rogers, Q. R. & Morris, J. G. (1978). *Journal of Nutrition* **108**, 1944.

Scott, P. P. (1984) In *Diseases of the Cat*, 2nd edn (ed. G. T. Wilkinson). Blackwell, Oxford.

Sturman, J. A., Gargano, A. D., Messing, J. M. & Imaki, H. (1986). *Journal of Nutrition*, **116**, 655–657.

Van den Broeck, A. H. M. & Thoday, K. L. (1986). *Journal of Small Animal Practice* **27**, 313.

CHAPTER 7

Diagnosis and Management of Hepatic Disorders

ALISON BLAXTER

INTRODUCTION

Conditions affecting the liver in the cat can be divided into two specific groups; primary hepatic diseases where pathological processes affect the liver alone, and generalized conditions affecting other systems and organs in which clinical signs of liver disease predominate.

Unlike the dog, hepatic cirrhosis associated with chronic liver insufficiency or insult is rare in the cat.

RECOGNITION OF HEPATIC DISEASE IN THE CAT

CLINICAL PRESENTATION

The most common presenting clinical signs of hepatic disease in the cat are jaundice and ascites, but these signs can be features of other conditions. For example, jaundice is commonly associated with feline infectious anaemia, caused by infection with the parasite *Haemobartonella felis*, and ascites may be a feature of bacterial peritonitis or, less commonly, of nephrotic syndrome or heart disease.

Although ascites and jaundice suggest liver disease, other
vague signs can predominate. The clinical history may include
insidious weight loss, intermittent anorexia, occasional vomiting, bouts of lethargy or depression and intermittent pyrexia.
Occasionally particular features may suggest a specific hepatic
disease. For example, polyphagia is a pronounced and distinctive feature of few conditions in the cat, but these include
lymphocytic cholangitis, hyperthyroidism and diabetes mellitus. Similarly, neurological signs of hepatic encephalopathy
in kittens associated with a congenital portosystemic shunt
are distinctive and rarely associated with any other condition.

If hepatic damage is part of a systemic disease there may
be signs associated with other systems. For example, in
an ascitic cat thoracic examination is essential and may
demonstrate pleural or, less commonly, pericardial effusions,
suggesting a diagnosis of feline infectious peritonitis. Hyperthyroidism can be associated with a diverse range of clinical
signs, including those of hepatic disease. Profound weight
loss, hyperactivity and signs associated with secondary hypertrophic cardiomyopathy may also be seen.

The major epidemiological features and presenting clinical
signs of the more common conditions are outlined in Tables
7.1–7.4 and the individual conditions are discussed in greater
detail below.

FURTHER INVESTIGATION

LABORATORY TESTS

As no single clinical sign is diagnostic for liver disease in the
cat, it is necessary to use laboratory tests in the majority of
cases.

Haematology

There are no consistent haematological abnormalities in feline
hepatic disease, but changes in haematology may suggest the
underlying aetiology. Cholangiohepatitis, as the result of
ascending bacterial infection, is commonly accompanied by a

Table 7.1 Primary liver diseases in the cat.

Cholangiohepatitis
Lymphocytic cholangitis
Neoplasia – FeLV associated lymphosarcoma
          – Primary bile duct carcinoma
          – Systemic mastocytosis
Primary congenital portosystemic shunt
Toxic hepatopathy

Table 7.2 Systemic conditions affecting the liver.

Feline infectious peritonitis
Hyperthyroidism
Hepatic lipidosis – Diabetes mellitus
                  – Hyperadrenocorticalism
                  – ? Idiopathic

Table 7.3 Differential diagnosis of jaundice in the cat.

Pre-hepatic or heamolytic	*Haemobartonella felis* infection (feline infectious anaemia) Autoimmune haemolytic anaemia FeLV associated haemolytic anaemias
Hepatocellular	Primary or secondary hepatic disease
Obstructive – intrahepatic	Primary hepatic disease involving neoplasia, hepatomegaly or intense inflammation
– extrahepatic	Chronic pancreatitis Pancreatic neoplasia Bile stones/bile duct obstruction Gall bladder trauma/rupture Obstruction of upper gastrointestinal tract

leucocytosis with neutrophilia and a left shift. Similarly, feline infectious peritonitis is characterized by non-regenerative anaemia and leucocytosis with lymphopenia, neutrophilia and a left shift. The pre-hepatic causes of jaundice should be identified by routine haematological examination and in the

Table 7.4 Differential diagnosis of ascites in the cat.

Primary hepatic disease
Feline infectious peritonitis
Bacterial peritonitis (secondary to penetrating skin wounds,
    gastrointestinal rupture or penetration, or as a postoperative
    complication)
Nephrotic syndrome (glomerulonephritis)
Heart disease – cardiomyopathy leading to congestive heart failure
Haemorrhage – traumatic, neoplastic
Bladder rupture
Biliary tract rupture
Chylous ascites

---

presence of anaemia, routine screening for *H. felis* with smears
stained with acridine orange, Giemsa or Wright's stain should
be performed.

Serum biochemistry

The liver enzyme alanine aminotransferase (ALT) will sensi-
tively indicate acute hepatocellular damage, while elevations
of serum alkaline phosphatase (SAP) and γ-glutamyl transferase (γ-GT) indicate cholestasis. Although SAP has been
routinely used to screen for evidence of liver damage it is
rapidly excreted by the kidney in cats and γ-GT may be a
much more useful measurement. Significant elevations of
these enzymes will indicate hepatic damage, but give no
indication as to cause, liver function or prognosis.

Where jaundice is present it is useful to consider the
proportion of conjugated (or water-soluble, direct reacting)
bilirubin and unconjugated (or indirect reacting) bilirubin.
Mixed jaundice would be expected in most primary hepatic
parenchymal diseases, and in those systemic conditions that
secondarily involve the liver. High proportions of conjugated
bilirubin indicate intra- or extra-hepatic biliary obstruction.
This can be associated with gross hepatomegaly in lymphocytic
cholangitis or advanced hepatic lymphosarcoma, or associated
with severe cholestasis such as in a suppurative cholangitis.

In dogs with chronic hepatic disease serum urea and
albumin are often markedly depressed, but as cirrhosis occurs
so rarely in the cat these abnormalities are very uncommon.

The immunological pathogenesis of two of the primary liver conditions in cats (lymphocytic cholangitis and feline infectious peritonitis) can make serum proteins, particularly globulin levels relevant. Both diseases can cause hypergammaglobulinaemia and globulin values greater than 50 g/litre, and often as high as 70 g/litre, are expected.

Evaluation of fasting serum ammonia concentration is of particular value in confirming hepatic encephalopathy in cases of suspected primary congenital portosystemic shunts. Secondary shunts related to portal hypertension in severe hepatic disease are extremely rare, and (not usually) extensive enough to produce clinical signs. The requirements for testing serum ammonia are exacting and samples must be separated within 30 min of sampling, analysed immediately, or frozen, and the results should be compared to a similarly starved control animal, evaluated at the same time. In general practice, local medical hospitals may be able to provide such a service, but otherwise this test should be performed at a referral centre with its own laboratory.

Radioimmune assay of serum bile acid concentrations may usefully test hepatobiliary function, particularly in relation to portosystemic anomalies, but, as yet it is not available in this country.

Assessment of hepatic function is at present made by monitoring the clearance of bromsulphthalein (BSP) from the circulation. The criteria for interpreting this test differ significantly in the dog and cat. In the cat, samples should be compared before the intravenous injection of 5 mg/kg BSP and 15 min after injection, rather than the standard evaluation at 30 min in the dog. There may be other dyes of greater reliability and significance, such as indocyanine green at 1.5 mg/kg, but these are not yet routinely used in Great Britain.

Serology to detect antibody titres to feline leukaemia virus and to feline infectious peritonitis virus may also be helpful in establishing the cause of hepatic disease and, consequently, the individual's prognosis.

The normal values for these parameters will vary between laboratories, and individual normal ranges should be consulted. The normal ranges used in the veterinary medicine laboratory at Bristol are given in Table 7.5.

Urinalysis

Cats have a low renal threshold for bilirubin but the presence of any bilirubinuria is abnormal and may indicate hepatic disease. Examination of urine sediment is of most use in confirming hepatic encephalopathy, as the presence of ammonium biurate crystals indicates hyperammonaemia associated with portosystemic shunting. Serum ammonia levels are highest following a meal and crystals are most prominent postprandially when urine is most likely to be alkaline. Oral bicarbonate may also help to induce alkaline urine.

Radiography

Radiography is of some value in the assessment of liver disease in cats. Lateral abdominal views will confirm the presence of ascites and should be repeated after abdominal paracentesis to assess hepatic size. Hepatic size can also be judged by administering 5–10 ml of liquid barium orally to outline the position of the gastric fundus.

Thoracic radiography may be indicated if hepatic disease is thought to be part of a systemic condition. For example, in feline infectious peritonitis pleural or pericardial effusions

Table 7.5 Normal values for liver tests in cats†. (From Blaxter, A. C. (1985). *Feline Hepatic Diseases*, Veterinary Annual.)

Alanine aminotransferase (ALT)	*16–44 iu/litre
Serum alkaline phosphatase (SAP)	*16–68 iu/litre
γ-Glutamyl transferase (γ-GT)	*< 10 iu/litre
Serum bilirubin (total)	< 5 umol/litre
Total protein	60–75 g/litre
Albumin	28–40 g/litre
Globulin	30–40 g/litre
Bromosulphthalein clearance (BSP)	< 10% at 15 min
Fasted serum ammonia	
	<100 mmol/litre (and comparison to control cat)
Whole blood clotting time*	3–5 min

*Performed at 37°C.
†From Bristol Veterinary Medicine Laboratory.

occur in at least 20% of cases that have ascites, and in hyperthyroidism, secondary hypertrophic cardiomyopathy with cardiomegaly and pulmonary oedema is common.

Abdominal paracentesis

Further investigation of hepatic disease often requires examination of fluid obtained by abdominal paracentesis. This can be performed with the cat in left lateral recumbency and a needle or catheter introduced through the ventral midline about one inch caudal to the umbilicus. Infiltration of the skin and abdominal muscle with local anaesthetic and sedation can be used, but is usually unnecessary.

Analysis of the fluid begins with an appreciation of its gross appearance, although this can be misleading, particularly in the differentiation of lymphocytic cholangitis and feline infectious peritonitis. In feline infectious peritonitis the fluid is classically viscous and straw coloured and may clot on standing. It has visually a globulin content in excess of 40 g/litre, but lymphocytic cholangitis can also be associated with a similarly globulin rich effusion.

Liver biopsy

This is often necessary to provide a definitive diagnosis for liver disease. However, the procedure for biopsy is not without risk and assessment of coagulation should be made before surgery. The easiest way to assess this in practice is to evaluate whole blood clotting time at 37°C although this is not a very sensitive test. Anaesthesia also presents difficulties in a patient with poor hepatic function.

Needle biopsy can be performed percutaneously under heavy sedation and analgesia or under general anaesthesia. There are disadvantages to this technique, for example, it does not permit direct visual assessment of liver disease, and haemorrhage is common after indirect biopsy. If it occurs it cannot be controlled as competently as at laparotomy.

Laparotomy under general anaesthesia is therefore preferable as it allows direct visualization of the liver and identification of any localized disease such as neoplasia or discrete lobar enlargement in lymphocytic cholangitis. Furthermore, other tissues in the abdominal cavity can be assessed, for example, for feline infectious peritonitis.

SPECIFIC HEPATIC CONDITIONS IN THE CAT

CHOLANGIOHEPATITIS

Ascending infection by enteric bacteria through the bile duct can result in an infective cholangiohepatitis. Clinical signs include intermittent pyrexia, and bouts of anorexia, vomiting, diarrhoea and lethargy with progressive weight loss and jaundice. Ascites is uncommon. Cats may resent anterior abdominal palpation and become severely dehydrated and depressed in the acute phases of the infection. The disease has been associated with cholelithiasis and pancreatitis but the frequency of this is unclear. If cholangiohepatitis is suspected, a diagnosis can be substantiated by haematological findings suggestive of acute bacterial infection, with moderate elevation of liver enzymes.

Hepatic biopsy is not usually necessary to confirm the diagnosis and, as the cat may be acutely ill with pressing needs for therapy it is seldom performed. However, histopathology demonstrates infiltration of the lumen of the bile tracts with neutrophils accompanied by an intense fibrotic periportal reaction.

Therapy involves correcting any fluid imbalance, giving appropriate antibiotics (such as the synthetic penicillins or potentiated sulphonamides, which are renal excreted and not hepatotoxic) and other supportive measures such as attention to diet. The use of corticosteroids in cholangiohepatitis is controversial but in the acute phases they may aid relief of inflammation. Prednisolone requires no hepatic activation so is usually recommended rather than prednisone.

The prognosis with prompt therapy is good, although recurrent bouts of infection may occur and antibiotics may have to be given for periods of one month and more.

PRIMARY CONGENITAL PORTOSYSTEMIC SHUNT

Portosystemic shunts are anomalous connections between the portal vein and systemic circulation. Shunting can occur either through a single congenital anomalous vein, or occur secondary to severe portal hypertension associated with chronic hepatic disease. A cirrhosis is rare in the cat, secondary portosystemic shunting is uncommon. As ammonia is normally degradated in the liver, shunting results in hyperammonaemia and this is associated with neurological abnormalities termed hepatic encephalopathy.

Cats with congenital portosystemic shunts are usually presented at 10 to 14 weeks old with dramatic hypersalivation (ptyalism). There may also be pupillary dilation, visual disturbances, behavioural changes (such as unprovoked aggression), ataxia and fits. The signs commonly associated with this abnormality in the dog, such as stunted growth, poor physical condition and intermittent vomiting and diarrhoea, are not usually recognized in the cat.

The only consistent biochemical finding is serum hyperammonaemia, as liver enzymes, BSP clearance, urea and albumin levels are usually normal. Urinalysis may reveal ammonium biurate crystals and if present these are diagnostic for hepatic encephalopathy. Most cases have livers of normal size on radiography.

The presence of a single congenital shunt is demonstrated by contrast portovenography (Fig. 7.1). Contrast medium, such as Conray "280" (RMB Animal Health), is introduced by catheter into a mesenteric vein and demonstrates the shunt bypassing the liver (Fig. 7.2). In the cat, these vessels are most commonly extrahepatic and accessible to surgical ligation. If partial ligation of the vessel is performed, normal blood flow through the liver can be encouraged and hyperammonaemia will be reduced with resolution of clinical signs. The few cases treated in this way have initially responded well, although recanalization has occurred when silk has been used as the suture material (Figs 7.3–7.5).

Whether or not surgery is completed, medical therapy should be initiated as soon as a diagnosis has been made, to try and reduce nitrogen waste levels. In some cases long term medical therapy alone may help to resolve clinical signs. This is achieved by reducing ammonia formation in the lower

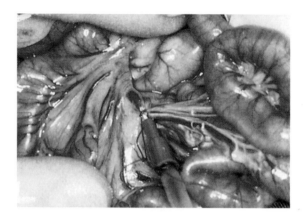

Fig. 7.1 In suspected hepatic encephalopathy, contrast portovenography is performed at laparotomy. An intravenous catheter is placed in a mesenteric vein, sutured loosely in position, and used to administer contrast media.

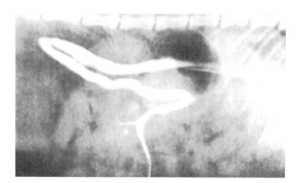

Fig. 7.2 Radiography after injection of contrast medium into a mesenteric vein in a case of congenital portosystemic shunt demonstrates a patent anomalous vessel shunting blood to the vena cava and bypassing the liver. In this cat the shunt involved a colonic vein.

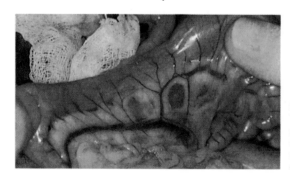

Fig. 7.3
The colonic vein could be seen grossly as a large dilated vessel draining blood from the mesenteric vein directly to the caudal vena cava.

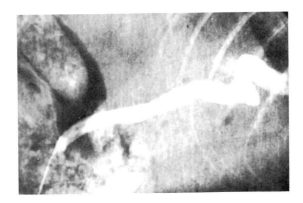

Fig. 7.4 A congenital portosystemic shunt may involve one of a number of vessels. In this radiograph an intrahepatic shunt has been visualized as a wide vessel communicating directly with the caudal venal cava. The configuration is typical of a patent ductus venosus.

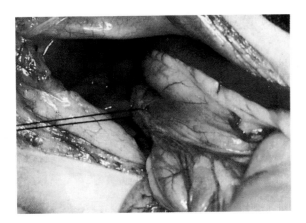

Fig. 7.5 Ligation of a portosystemic shunt can be performed at laparotomy after contrast portovenography. Here a gastroduodenal vein is being ligated. Silk may not be the most suitable material for ligation as recanalization has occurred in some cases 12–24 months postoperatively.

gastrointestinal tract through limitation of protein intake and by administering oral neomycin and lactulose.

LYMPHOCYTIC CHOLANGITIS

This primary hepatic disorder was first described in 1982. It involves an intense lymphocytic infiltration and proliferation of bile ducts which progresses to lobular fibrosis, with gross distortion of liver architecture (Figs 7.6 and 7.7). The clinical syndrome occurs most commonly in cats less than 5 years old in contrast to bacterial cholangiohepatitis which appears to be more common in older cats. The history usually includes polyphagia, intermittent vomiting or regurgitation, progressive abdominal distension with ascites and hepatomegaly, and jaundice. However, despite these changes the cats are often bright, alert and apyrexic. The hepatomegaly may be palpable as diffuse enlargement, or it may involve single lobes or discrete portions of the liver.

Laboratory examination will give evidence of cholestasis with the most marked changes being dramatic elevations of conjugated bilirubin, serum alkaline phosphatase and γ-glutamyl transferase. Both ascitic fluid and serum have high globulin levels and haematology may demonstrate non-regenerative anaemia, lymphopenia and neutrophilia. These findings are very similar to those made in feline infectious peritonitis.

Definitive diagnosis is made by histopathological examination of a liver biopsy (Figs 7.8 and 7.9). The intense lymphocytic infiltration and bile duct proliferation suggests an autoimmune aetiology. Therapy with immunosuppressive doses of prednisolone can produce dramatic resolution of clinical signs, hepatomegaly and biochemical abnormalities over a period of 4–12 weeks. Concurrent supportive therapy with abdominal paracentesis, diuresis, and appropriate diet are also indicated. The duration of prednisolone therapy required varies between cases. Some require continual low dose therapy while others enter remission after 8–12 weeks, although recurrent bouts of disease can occur.

TOXIC HEPATOPATHY

The inability of the cat's liver to deal with many routinely used drugs and household substances is well known. One of the primary reasons for this is that the feline liver cannot efficiently conjugate and excrete some toxins so that tissues are exposed for longer. Hepatocellular damage has been

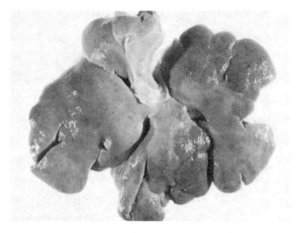

Fig. 7.6 Liver demonstrating gross appearance of lymphocytic cholangitis. The liver is enlarged and firm with nodularity of the capsular surface and exaggerated lobular markings.

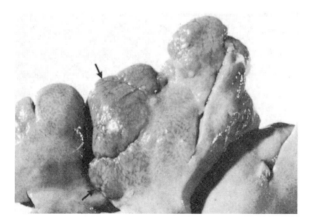

Fig. 7.7 Close up of liver lymphocytic cholangitis demonstrating nodularity of the capsular surface and abnormal tortuous vessels (arrow). (From Lucke and Davies (1984) *Journal of Small Animal Practice* **25**, 249, with kind permission.)

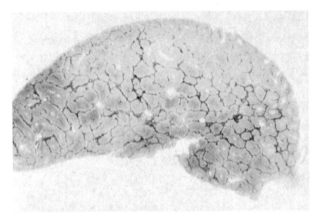

Fig. 7.8 Section of liver with lymphocytic cholangitis showing complete and incomplete monolobular fibrosis. Haematoxylin – van Giesen × 7. (From Lucke and Davies (1984) *Journal of Small Animal Practice* 25, 249, with kind permission.)

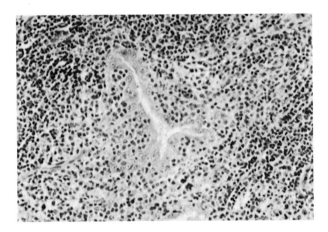

Fig. 7.9 In lymphocytic cholangitis a dense lymphocytic exudate encircles and penetrates damaged bile duct epithelium (Haematoxylin and eosin × 195). (From Lucke and Davies (1984) *Journal of Small Animal Practice* 25, 249, with kind permission.)

associated with many hepatotoxins including the phenolic disinfectants and oestrogens.

The clinical and biochemical findings are non-specific but often include jaundice, chronic weight loss and lethargy without ascites. No specific therapy is usually available and treatment centres around supportive measures with identification of any possible toxins and their withdrawal.

HEPATIC NEOPLASIA

Neoplasis is an uncommon feline hepatic disease. Lymphosarcoma related to feline leukaemia virus infection is most frequently found. Systemic mastocytosis also occurs but is uncommon, resulting in diffuse mast cell neoplasms in liver and spleen. Primary hepatic carcinomas also occur, often involving the bile ducts. The clinical signs in hepatic neoplasia are often vague and when recognized, the disease may be well advanced. Pancreatic carcinoma is probably more frequently a cause of obstructive jaundice in the cat.

FELINE INFECTIOUS PERITONITIS

Feline infectious peritonitis, first described in the UK in 1970, is caused by infection with a coronavirus and can involve with a variety of signs, some of which are hepatic. The disease may occur in all breeds, ages and sexes of cat but there is an increased prevalence in oriental breeds and in those cats under 2 years or over 10 years.

The initial phase of the condition (which can last up to 3 months) is characterized by clinical signs which are vague and may be prolonged. These include inappetence, lethargy, anaemia and fever, occasionally with signs of upper respiratory tract infection. Two major forms of the condition can follow. The clinical signs of the "wet", effusive, form include ascites, dyspnoea and tachypnoea associated with pleural and, or, pericardial effusion, jaundice, weight loss and wasting, persistent anorexia, depression and anaemia.

In the non-effusive or "dry" form, anorexia and depression persist, but signs in other systems occur without ascites. The pattern of clinical signs is related to the pyogranulomatous lesions in various tissues and signs of hepatic disease with jaundice, but without gross ascites, may be prominent.

The most significant findings with serum biochemistry are hyperglobulinaemia (greater than 40 g/litre and often greater than 60 g/litre) and moderate elevation of liver enzymes. Non-regenerative anaemia, leucocytosis with left shift and lymphopenia may be demonstrated by haematology.

Histopathology of liver, peritoneum, pleura, meninges, kidneys, etc. will confirm the typical and characteristic pyo-

Table 7.6 Major historical and clinical features of the more common hepatic disorders in the cat. (From Blaxter, A. C. (1985). *Feline Hepatic Disease, Veterinary Annual*.)

Condition	Epidemiology	Onset	Most common presenting clinical features
Cholangiohepatitis	All breeds/ages/sexes	Acute with recurrent bouts	Recurrent pyrexia, abdominal pain, vomiting, lethargy, anorexia, dehydration, jaundice
Lymphocytic cholangitis	Most common in cats < 5 years	Insidious	Hepatomegaly, ascites, jaundice, polyphagia, sporadic vomiting or regurgitation
Toxic hepatitis	All breeds/ages/sexes Known access to hepatotoxins	Acute or insidious	Acute jaundice and abdominal pain or insidious weight loss with jaundice
Primary portosystemic shunt	All breeds/sexes Onset usually at 10–14 weeks but cases in adults reported	Acute and dramatic	Ptyalism and signs of hepatic encephalopathy (pupillary dilatation, visual disturbance, character changes, ataxia, fits)
Neoplasia	Most common in older cats > 10 years May be an association with FeLV infection	Insidious	Hepatomegaly
Feline infectious peritonitis	All breeds/ages/sexes but greatest incidence in Orientals < 2 years or > 10 years	Often insidious	Persistent pyrexia, lethargy, anorexia, leading to ascites, jaundice, pleural effusion
Hyperthyroidism	All breeds/sexes. Most common > 6 years, especially around 10 years	Insidious	Chronic weight loss, polyphagia, hyperactivity, palpable thyroid nodules, tachycardia

granulomatous lesions. No therapy is possible and as the course of the disease can be protracted and distressing euthanasia is indicated.

HYPERTHYROIDISM

This is a recently recognized clinical disorder and is one of the major causes of weight loss and wasting in cats over 10 years old. Clinical signs are related to increased levels of circulating thyroid hormones (primarily T4, and T3) associated with functioning neoplasms of one or both thyroid glands. These are usually bilateral benign adenomas, although occasionally adenocarcinomas occur.

Clinical signs include dramatic weight loss, polyphagia, polydipsia, hyperactivity, behavioural changes (such as increased aggression), vomiting or regurgitation, diarrhoea, seborrhoea and a poor, greasy, matted coat (lack of grooming), jaundice and sometimes signs related to secondary cardiomy-opathy. A clinical diagnosis can be substantiated by finding palpably enlarged thyroid glands and by serum biochemistry. Increased liver enzymes will demonstrate non-specific hepato-cellular damage and T4 and, or, T3 levels will be grossly elevated. If auscultation, radiology and ECG suggest cardiomy-opathy, these will also suggest hyperthyroidism.

Therapy can be very successful. It involves surgical, medical or chemical ablation of the functioning thyroid neoplasms.

HEPATIC LIPIDOSIS

Diabetes mellitus and hyperadrenocorticalism, although comparatively rare in the cat, may induce signs that are associated with fatty degeneration of the liver. In extreme cases, hepato-megaly and jaundice may occur but disease is most often indicated only by elevation of liver enzymes, indicating mild hepatocellular, damage and cholestasis. The signs of the underlying endocrine disease will predominate, with polydip-sia, polyuria, polyphagia, weight loss, and, in the case of diabetes mellitus, glycosuria.

Hepatic lipidosis has also been described as a primary disease in the cat, related to obesity and stress, with elevated

Table 7.7 Diagnostic features of the more common conditions of the liver in the cat.

Condition	Haematology, serum biochemistry, examination of fluid obtained by abdominal paracentesis	Radiography	Hepatic biopsy
Cholangiohepatitis	Leucocytosis with neutrophilia and left shift suggestive of bacterial infection	Non-specific. Ascites uncommon	Intra-luminal infiltration of the bile tracts by neutrophils with evidence of fibrosis and neutrophil infiltration periportally
Lymphocytic cholangitis	Non-regenerative anaemia, lymphopenia, and neutrophilia Moderate to high elevation of liver enzymes, particularly SAP and γ-GT. Mixed jaundice. Ascitic fluid also high in globulin, straw coloured and viscous	Generalized hepatomegaly or discrete enlargement of one hepatic lobe. Ascites	Lymphocytic infiltration and proliferation of bile ducts progressing to lobular fibrosis
Toxic hepatitis	Non-specific – elevation of liver enzymes	Ascites uncommon	Hepatocellular degeneration
Primary portosystemic shunt	Hyperammonaemia, often without other indications of hepatic disease. BSP clearance commonly normal	Occasionally cases demonstrate hepatic atrophy on X-ray.	Usually normal although absence of portal triads has been reported

		Contrast portal venography will confirm a functional anomalous portosystemic shunt	
Neoplasia	Non-specific elevation of liver enzymes	Hepatomegaly or discrete enlargement of a liver lobe	Neoplastic infiltration
Feline infectious peritonitis	Non-regenerative anaemia, leucocytosis with lymphopenia and neutrophilia Hypergammaglobulinaemia and globulin rich, straw-coloured, viscous abdominal fluid. Positive serological titre to coronaovirus	20% of cases with ascites also have pleural and, or, pericardial effusions	Pyogranulomatous lesions on peritoneum, pleura and within tissues, e.g. liver, kidney, brain, lung
Hyperthyroidism	Non-specific moderate elevation of liver enzymes Elevated thyroxine (T4) levels	Secondary hypertrophic cardiomyopathy common (cardiomegaly, pleural oedema)	Non-specific

Table 7.8 Suggested treatment and prognosis for some liver diseases in the cat.

Condition	Therapy	Prognosis
Cholangiohepatitis	14–21 days antibiotic therapy (synthetic penicillins, potentiated sulphonamides), fluid therapy and intensive nursing in the acute phases, followed by supportive therapy (vitamins, encouraging appetite, appropriate diet) prednisolone (0.5 mg/kg) in acute stages	Good, although recurrent bouts can occur
Lymphocytic cholangitis	Immunosuppressant doses of prednisolone over 12 weeks (2 mg/kg daily reducing to low dose alternate day therapy). Supportive therapy – paracentesis, diuresis, fluids, vitamins, appropriate diet	Some cats respond extremely well to therapy while others require intermittent therapy
Toxic hepatitis	Identify and eliminate source of toxin supportive therapy	Variable

Primary portosystemic shunt	Medical – low volume/high quality protein diet (e.g. boiled rice mixed 50/50 with lean white meat, cottage cheese), lactulose orally (1 ml three times daily "Duphalac" Duphar) neomycin orally. Surgery – partial ligation of extrahepatic shunt	Guarded – a good response has been gained after surgery
Neoplasia	Hepatic neoplasia commonly indicates an advanced and systemic condition such as feline leukaemia virus infection or mastocytosis. No treatment is indicated	Hopeless
Feline infectious peritonitis	No specific therapy possible	Hopeless
Hyperthyroidism	The treatment of choice is surgical removal of the affected gland(s). Pre-operative management of cardiomyopathy – propranolol (2.5–5 mg three times daily), reduce stress. Propylthiouracil, carbimazole or potassium iodide orally to medically reduce T4 levels pre-operatively	Good
Hepatic lipidosis	Related to the specific condition	Dependent on underlying metabolic derangement

levels of serum SAP. However, it is very poorly documented as a distinct clinical condition and its relationship to endocrine disorders has not been clarified.

CONCLUSION

The numerous hepatic diseases of the cat, summarized in Tables 7.6–7.8, present challenges to the small animal practitioner in diagnosis and management. The most common presenting clinical signs of feline hepatic diseases are jaundice and ascites, but these signs can be associated with disease in other systems, and the history and presenting abnormalities in cats with liver disease are often vague and non-specific. Management of the different hepatic diseases in the cat also varies considerably, according to specific aetiology, adding to the importance of accurate diagnosis.

CHAPTER 8

Feline Dysautonomia

ALISON BLAXTER AND TIM GRUFFYDD-JONES

INTRODUCTION

Feline dysautonomia was first recognized in Great Britain during the winter of 1981–1982. In 1984 two detailed reports were published describing the clinical features, diagnosis, management and pathological abnormalities of the syndrome and included some brief epidemiological observations (Rochlitz, 1984; Sharp et al., 1984). Changes are now apparent in both the pattern and appearance of the condition.

EPIDEMIOLOGY AND AETIOLOGY

Cases have been reported from all areas of the UK and Scandinavia. One of the most puzzling features of the disease has been the sudden and dramatic appearance of the condition in these well defined areas. Only few and sporadic cases have been reported elsewhere, including the USA and the United Arab Emirates, but often in British households or in cats of British origin.

It is difficult to assess the incidence of a particular disease in a referral centre and a large prospective study would be necessary to assess accurately the incidence of dysautonomia in the feline population. However, there has been a striking decrease in the number of cases seen in this clinic over the past 2 years. Similarly, many veterinary surgeons in practice report a considerable reduction in the incidence of the syndrome since an initial peak in the 2 years following the first reports. It is interesting that a similar and recent fall in the incidence of the syndrome is thought to have occurred in Scandinavia following an initial dramatic peak.

As the aetiology of feline dysautonomia remains undetermined, the relevance of these apparent recent reductions in incidence and the restricted geographical distributions is unclear. The strong resemblance of the clinical signs, histopathological findings and the similar geographical pattern to those characteristic of equine grass disease is also puzzling. The significance of this remains unknown.

Practitioners have reported both temporal and seasonal clustering of cases. Although cases initially referred here appeared to be most frequent during the autumn and winter, this trend has not continued.

Rochlitz (1984) reported no sex predisposition in the cases seen initially at Langford and reported an age range of 15 weeks to 11 years with the majority of cases being in young adults. Similar findings are apparent on examination of the cases seen subsequently at this clinic. Of the 30 cases seen here from 1983 to 1985 the majority of cases were under 3 years of age, five were under 6 months, and the age of cases ranged from 6 weeks to 10 years.

Investigation of the lifestyle and other epidemiological features of affected cats has continued, but has failed to reveal any factor common to all cases. There continues to be no evidence for an infectious agent. Where the syndrome occurs in a multicat household, usually only one individual is affected. However, if more than one cat develops the condition they are often related. The significance of this observation to the aetiology remains unclear.

CLINICAL SIGNS

In many of our cases there was a "prodromal" period which occurred for 24 h to 4 days before the onset of definitive clinical signs and this has also been reported by previous authors. Cats may show signs of mild upper respiratory tract infection with serous ocular and nasal discharge, and in others diarrhoea is seen initially. One of the most interesting features of the condition is that in a multicat household other cats may show these signs while only one individual may subsequently develop further signs of feline dysautonomia.

The major clinical signs principally represent severe damage to both parasympathetic and sympathetic branches of the autonomic nervous system. More common clinical signs are given in Tables 8.1 and 8.2. The frequency of these clinical signs in previous and recent cases is indicated in Table 8.3.

A comparison of the clinical signs shown by the cases reported in 1983 with those seen between 1983 and 1985 (see

Table 8.1 Common clinical signs in feline dysautonomia.

Severe anorexia
Depression
Vomiting
Regurgitation
Dysphagia associated with megaoesophagus
Small intestinal stasis
Lower gastrointestinal tract stasis with constipation
Dry oral, ocular and nasal mucosae with reduced lacrimation and
    salivation
Bilateral protrusion of the nictitating membranes
Dehydration
Bilaterally dilated pupils with sluggish light responses
Photophobia
Bradycardia – less than 90 beats/min

Less common signs include

Skin fragility
Dysuria with urinary retention
Anisocoria
Syncope or collapse
Ataxia associated with poor hindlimb proprioception

Table 8.2 Incidence of major clinical signs in dysautonomia cases.

Number of major clinical signs	Number of cases
1	0
2	2
3	8
4	10
5	8

The five major clinical signs are:

Regurgitation/demonstrable
  megoesophagus
Dilated pupils
Constipation
Depression
Dry nasal ocular or oral mucosae

Table 8.3 Frequency of clinical signs.

	Early Bristol cases*	Glasgow cases†	Recent Bristol cases
Number of cases	46	40	28
Clinical signs (% of cases)			
Dilated pupils	93	90	57
Megoesophagus	89	92	64
Regurgitation/vomiting	87	82	64
Dry nose	85	95	43
Protrusion of nictitating membranes	80	71	36
Constipation	78	95	54
Dry mouth	76	69	39
Depression	60	100	64
Dysphagia	98	NR	43
Anorexia	33	NR	53
Bradycardia	23	59	18
Dysuria	17	18	39
Ataxia	7	14	4
Faecal incontinence	7	20	11
Recovery	22	30	50

NR Not recorded.
*Rochlitz (1984).
†Sharp *et al.* (1984).

Table 8.3) demonstrates some interesting differences. The most striking observation is that there has been a marked reduction in frequency of the clinical signs most commonly encountered previously. This substantiates the impression of many veterinary surgeons in practice that not only the incidence but also the severity of the disease is declining. It is therefore now of importance to recognize the possibility of feline dysautonomia in cases with only two or three of the major clinical signs.

DIFFERENTIAL DIAGNOSIS

In its "classical form" it is difficult to confuse dysautonomia with any other condition in the cat. However, now that less severe expressions of the disease are commonly seen, it is relevant to consider other diagnoses, particularly those that cause persistent regurgitation or vomiting and those that produce ocular lesions involving pupillary size. For example, a partial gastrointestinal obstruction, particularly in the lower small intestine will produce persistent vomiting, and radiographic evidence of lower gastrointestinal stasis.

AIDS TO DIAGNOSIS

The only useful aids to diagnosis after detailed clinical examination are radiography and ocular examination. Megoesophagus can usually be demonstrated on lateral radiographs of the thorax and neck and outlined by the administration of 5–10 ml of liquid barium by mouth. Immediate and 10 min films will show pooling and retention of barium either along the whole of the oesophagus or in discrete areas. (In normal animals, immediate films should show only streaky retention of barium on the oesophageal mucosa. At 10 min this should have disappeared.)

Estimation of tear secretion using Schirmer tear test papers may aid a subjective assessment of poor tear flow and salivation in a suspected case.

TREATMENT

Rochlitz (1984) discussed the management of dysautonomia comprehensively and approach to treatment in this clinic has remained very similar. The two main aspects of treatment are non-specific supportive therapy and specific treatment with parasympathomimetics. This is outlined in the Tables 8.4 and 8.5.

PROGNOSIS

The prognosis for cats with dysautonomia appears to have improved in that 50% of affected cats seen at this clinic between October of 1983 and 1985 survived. Earlier reports indicated recovery rates of 20 and 30%. Improved management of the syndrome resulting from increased experience, and the apparent reduction in severity, have probably both contributed to the more favourable prognosis. Persistent, unresponsive anorexia, extensive megoesophagus and dysuria remain indicators of a poor prognosis.

Cats which survive the initial episode of dysautonomia commonly suffer from further problems in the future. The most common of these are recurrent gastrointestinal problems. Affected cats may show recurrent constipation, which is

Table 8.4 Non-specific therapy for dysautonomia.

Fluid therapy	Intravenous, subcutaneous, intraperitoneal, oral
Appetite stimulation	Corticosteroids, multivitamins, vitamin B_{12}, anabolic steroids
Enemas	Glycerol and water, liquid paraffin and glycerol, "Microlax" (Smith, Kline and French)
Oral laxatives	Liquid paraffin, "Katalax" (C-Vet)
Dietary management	Postural feeding of liquid (soup consistency) foods at body temperature
Steam inhalation	Stimulates salivation and lacrimation
Warmth	
Antibiotics	

Table 8.5 Specific therapy in dysautonomia – parasympathomimetics.

Drug	Dose	Contraindications/comments
Pilocarpine 1% eye drops Physostigmine 0.5% eye drops	1 or 2 drops twice a day	Dilution occasionally necessary when over-stimulation occurs (hypersalivation, abdominal straining). Useful in cases of persistent regurgitation. (Give 5–20 min before feeding)
Bethanecol chloride (Myotonine Glenwood)	2.5 mg orally two or six times daily	Do not use in cases of bradycardia (< 100 beats/min). Use with great care in combination with other parasympathomimetics
Danthron (Dorbanex Forte suspension; Riker)	2–5 ml daily	Acid laxative and parasympathomimetic. Very useful in the control of lower gut stasis. Can be used freely with other parasympathomimetics

usually most satisfactorily managed with periodic administration of danthron (Dorbanex Forte suspension; Riker). The development of faecal incontinence can be a late complication and can be very difficult to manage successfully, although it can be associated with overdosing with parasympathomimetics. Megoesophagus appears to persist but in most surviving cats regurgitation or vomiting becomes occasional. In those cats with persistent regurgitation, dietary management with the provision of a liquidized posturally-fed diet is often the most successful control measure. Some surviving cats retain a fastidious appetite while others may require two or three times their original food intake to retain normal bodyweight. A proportion of cases never completely recover their previous bodily condition. Pupil size and pupillary light response may or may not improve.

Occasionally recovered cats will show an acute recurrence of signs. Such signs are not usually as severe as those seen in the initial stages of the disease and will usually respond well to short-term therapy. Several of our surviving cats have subsequently developed peculiar complications of apparent neurological origin such as blindness, disorientation and collapse. It is not clear whether these complications are related to earlier episodes of dysautonomia although in one case the pronounced bradycardia may have been a factor.

REFERENCES

Rochlitz, I. (1984). *Journal of Small Animal Practice* **25**, 587.
Sharp, N. J. H., Nash, A. S. & Griffiths, I. R. (1984). *Journal of Small Animal Practice* **25**, 599.

CHAPTER 9

Ocular Disease

PETER BEDFORD

CONGENITAL DEFECTS AND DISEASES

Feline congenital ocular abnormalities are relatively uncommon but structural defects and disease involving the whole eye, eyelids, nasolacrimal duct system, uveal tract, lens, retina and optic nerve have all been reported (Peiffer, 1982). Unfortunately the cat is not subjected to the same extensive eye examination and control schemes that exist for dogs. Such schemes for the cat could reveal the true incidence of congenital disease and prove helpful in indicating any breed predisposition.

THE GLOBE

Abnormalities related to the gross development of the eye are rarely seen. In anophthalmia the eyelids have developed and there is a normal palpebral fissure but a recognizable globe is not present; in microphthalmia the globe is present but remains underdeveloped to varying degrees. Both conditions may be unilateral or bilateral, and where slight microphthalmia only is present the eye may be capable of normal vision.Careful assessment is required before the prognosis is given.

Buphthalmia or congenital glaucoma is similarly of low incidence, the eye(s) being enlarged and blind at the time of birth.

Congenital convergent strabismus (squint) or esotropia is seen most commonly in the Siamese and is probably inherited as an autosomal recessive trait. The underlying cause is deficient development of the subcortical visual pathways. Retinal function remains apparently normal and surgical correction of the squint by repositioning the lateral and medial rectus muscles on the sclera is possible but seldom proves necessary.

Similar deficiency of the subcortical visual pathways is probably responsible for the congenital nystagmus also seen in the Siamese breed. Although the appearance of the cat is often distressing to the owner, the condition does not seem to affect functional vision.

THE EYELIDS

Congenital conditions can inolve the eyelid and are important because of possible associated corneal disease. Persistent ankyloblepharon, in which the lid margins remain united after birth may be associated with neonatal keratoconjunctivitis (ophthalmia neanatorum). Symblepharon (Fig. 9.1), permanent corneal opacity, keratoconjunctivitis sicca and even loss of the eye may occur unless the condition is relieved. The lid margins must be separated and appropriate antibiotic therapy administered.

Most congenital symblepharon is related to necnatal inflammatory disease and adhesions between the bulbar and palpebral conjunctival tissues can influence palpebral mobility or effect permanent protrusion of the membrana nictitans. Adhesions between the conjunctiva and the cornea can impair vision or render the patient blind.

Surgical correction of symblepharon at any age is difficult. Readhesions tend to occur despite corticosteroid therapy and the possible use of a hydrophilic contact lens as a physical barrier between the dissected surfaces during healing.

Bilateral agenesis or coloboma (Fig.9.2) of the temporal part of the upper eyelid occurs most frequently in the domestic short-haired cat. "Coloboma" means an absence of ocular

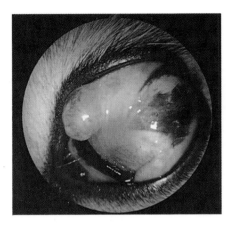

Fig. 9.1
Congenital symblepharon, the conjunctival
tissues covering the whole corneal surface. Left
eye.

tissue and eyelid colobomas can occur with iridal and posterior
segmental colobomas. This association is not understood, as
some iridal and choroidal colobomas are considered to be
inherited as autosomal dominant traits while the eyelid defect
is believed to be non-hereditable. The absence of a functional
eyelid margin means that the remnant eyelid tissue is fused
with the dorsolateral bulbar conjunctiva and episcleral tissues.
In this area a conjunctival sac does not exist and subsequent
corneal disease is related to exposure and an inability to
spread the precorneal tear film. Irritation caused by the
contacting eyelid hair can be countered by entropion surgery
but correction is best achieved by a sliding facial skin graft
(Bistner *et al.*, 1977) or a lateral canthal based pedicle graft
from the lower lid to fill the defect and provide a partially
functional lid margin (Bedford, 1980).

Neonatal entropion can be bilateral or unilateral and most
commonly involves the lower eyelid and the Persian breed.
The classical signs are trigeminal irritation or pain. Correction
by the Hotz-Celsus skin or skin/muscle technique should be
effected before severe keratoconjunctivitis and corneal erosion
can occur.

Dermoids involving the cornea, conjunctiva and eyelid
are uncommon but they should be removed by superficial
keratectomy to relieve irritation and restore vision.

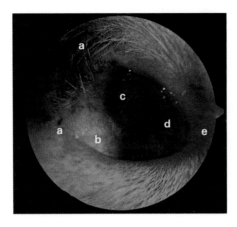

Fig. 9.2
Coloboma of the right upper lid. Seven-month-old DSH. a, Extent of the coloboma; b, bulbar conjunctiva overlying the sclera; c, iris; d, pupil; e, medial canthus.

THE LACRIMAL SYSTEM

The lacrimal system may demonstrate both congenital defect and be affected by congenital disease. Keratoconjunctivitis sicca caused by the destruction of the lacrimal gland or occlusion of its excretory ducts and due to neonatal inflammatory disease has already been mentioned. Epiphora may result from the occlusion of the lower lacrimal punctum, the lower canaliculus and/or the nasolacrimal duct, related to the same neonatal inflammatory disease processes.

Neonatal epiphora due to nasolacrimal duct or canaliculus aplasia is unusual but both stenosis of these structures and aplasia of the lower lacrimal punctum occur rather more frequently. Stenosis of the duct or canaliculus is most commonly seen in the Persian and is simply demonstrated by the absence of nasal drainage by gravity of fluorescein solution applied to the cornea. Forced nasal drainage of a fluorescein solution can be effected using a blunted 25 gauge hypodermic needle and syringe, but it should be remembered that such drainage does not equate with normal drainage produced by blinking and capillary flow.

Epiphora due to aplasia of the lacrimal punctum can occur in any breed of cat. In the absence of stenosis elsewhere in the drainage system, the lower canaliculus may be opened lengthwise and fashioned into a "gutter" to assist in drainage of the lacrimal lake and possibily relieve the overflow.

THE UVEAL TRACT

Congenital defects involving the uveal tract are uncommon in the cat. Anterior uveal cysts are benign pigmented fluid-filled spherical swellings usually located at the pupillary margins but may break free and gravitate into the ventral pcrtion of the anterior chamber.

Persistent pupillary membranes are remnants of the tunica vasculosa lentis. They may be seen usually as pigmented strands of tissue within the pupillary aperture or adhering to the cornea or the lens. This adherence may be marked by opacity but vision is seldom impaired.

THE LENS

Congenital cataract is also uncommon but cpacities of the anterior capsular and subcapsular regions of the lens may occur in associaticn with persistent pupillary membranes. Posterior polar cataract (Fig. 9.3) may be due to the persistence of hyaloid blood vessels. Both types of cataract are usually non-progressive and do not interfere with functional vision.

Maternal prenatal systemic infection, fetal ocular infection and inadequate nutrition during pregnancy may cause congenital nuclear cataracts (Fig. 9.4) which are usually non-progressive but may impair vision considerably because of their size and position within the lens. The possibility of inheritance should be considered, particularly when the lesion is seen in several related cats.

THE RETINA AND OPTIC NERVE

The feline fundus is rarely affected by congenital defect but optic nerve hypoplasia, disc colobomas and retinal dysplasia associated with both maternal and neonatal systemic diseases have been recorded.

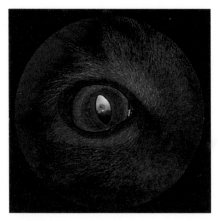

Fig. 9.3
Posterior polar cataract in a 6-month-old DSH. Right
eye before mydriasis.

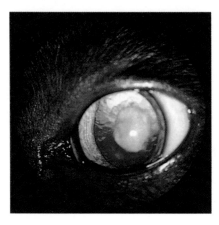

Fig. 9.4
Nuclear cataract in a 5-month-old DSH. Left eye,
following mydriasis.

ACQUIRED OCULAR DISEASE

THE ORBIT

Orbital trauma, infection and neoplasia can be responsible for
proptosis, protrusion of the membrana nictitans, lagophthalmos, exposure keratitis and blindness due to optic nerve
damage.

Orbital trauma is commonly accompanied by subconjunctival and retrobulbar haemorrhage (Fig. 9.5). Prolapse of the

globe can be more difficult to manage surgically than in the dog because of an increased globe to orbit size ratio. Ocular venostasis and optic nerve damage represent the most important factors in prognosis and as such the duration of the prolapse is critical.

Tarsorrhaphy using a mattress suture pattern for 14 days will maintain the eye in the orbit. Post-operative diuretic and corticosteroid therapy is essential but globe deviation, due to extraocular muscle damage, oculomotor nerve damage, and blindness are frequent sequelae.

Orbital infection is usually associated with the presence of retrobulbar foreign body material and periapical infection of the upper molar teeth. Pain usually prevents mastication and, though antibiosis may prove effective, drainage of the orbit can be necessary. Occasionally, this can be done through the upper lid but additional blunt dissection from the oral cavity to the orbit behind the last tooth will provide a more persistent drainage route.

Orbital neoplasia represents the significant differential diagnosis but pain is not usually manifest and chronic optic neuropraxia may be indicated by mydriasis, an absence of the direct pupillary light reflex, retinal blood vessel congestion and papilloedema. Surgical exploration of the orbit (Harvey, 1977) is possible and biopsy gives definitive diagnosis.

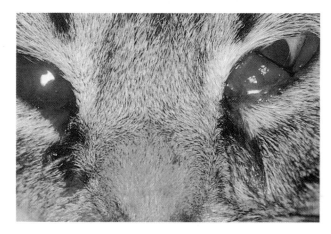

Fig. 9.5
Subconjunctival haemorrhage associated with orbital trauma.

THE EYELIDS

Acquired disease of the eyelids is due to trauma, inflammation, infection and neoplasia and there may be accompanying or subsequent corneal disease.

Blepharitis, inflammation of eyelid tissue, is most commonly seen with acute conjunctivitis and may be complicated by self-trauma and infection. Treatment is effected by attention to cause and the appropriate antibiotic and corticosteroid therapy. *Notoedres cati* and *Microsporum canis* can cause blepharitis and should be treated appropriately.

Wounds involving eyelid margins must be repaired to avoid cicatricial distortion and subsequent conjunctival and corneal disease. Entropion may occur and any part of the eyelid margin can be involved (Fig. 9.6).

Chronic conjunctivitis is the other cause of cicatricial entropion and may occur bilaterally with both upper and lower eyelids affected. With entropion the movement of hair against the cornea causes trigeminal irritation and hyperlacrimation; tear film overflow and blepharospasm are constantly present. Keratitis and superficial corneal erosion may result if the defect is not corrected.

Blepharospasm itself will increase the degree of entropion but unrelieved blepharospasm can produce a secondary entropion. While cicatricial entropion needs correction, entropion which is secondary to corneal disease rarely requires eyelid surgery. The blepharospasm should be broken by using a

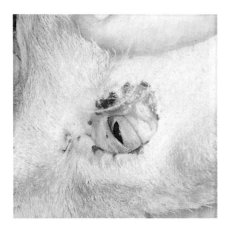

Fig. 9.6
Ectropion of the left upper eyelid due to localized chronic inflammation.

membrana flap to cover the cornea during the healing period. Once trigeminal irritation has ceased the entropion is invariably relieved.

Ectropion is unusual in the cat but may occur as the result of eyelid trauma or cicatrization associated with chronic inflammation. Any part of the eyelid can be involved, significant distortion being most easily achieved away from the medial canthus. Conjunctival exposure with conjunctivitis, lagophthalmos and exposure keratitis may also be present. A V to Y plasty may provide adequate correction, but techniques of resection at the lateral canthus and sliding skin grafts (Bedford, 1980) can prove useful.

Eyelid neoplasia is relatively common in the cat, the major tumour being squamous cell carcinoma (Fig. 9.7) The margo-intermarginalis is the usual site of origin but the membrana nictitans and cornea may also be primarily involved. Removal by excision or cryosurgery can be successful providing there is an early diagnosis. Extensive tumour formation can be treated by combining excision with subsequent radiation therapy.

CONJUNCTIVITIS

Conjunctivitis is a common condition in the cat but the aetiology often proves difficult to establish. Conjunctival

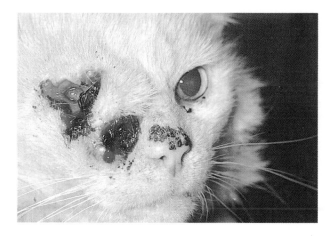

Fig. 9.7
Long standing squamous cell carcinoma involving the whole of the right palpebral fissure and facial skin in a 7-year-old white DSH.

scrapes and biopsies for virus isolation, bacterial culture and histology can help, the tissue being taken from the anterior aspect of the membrana nictitans or the palpebral conjunctiva at the base of the lower lid under local anaesthesia.

Acute conjunctivitis may be characterized by chemosis, gross hyperaemia and discomfort whereas chronic disease may be indicated by nothing more than a slight sero-mucous discharge and little hyperaemia.

The discharge which accompanies a conjunctivitis can vary considerably in quantity and type, the serous, mucous, or purulent characteristics indicating the severity of the response and possible bacterial involvement. The presence of foreign body material, chemical irritation and local trauma are most often associated with unilateral conjunctivitis. (Fig. 9.8) Bilateral conjunctivitis is usually associated with systemic disease.

Most conjunctivitis is seen in association with viral upper respiratory tract (URT) disease and herpesvirus, calicivirus or reovirus may be responsible. It is suggested that herpesvirus is probably the most common cause of conjunctivitis which accompanies URT disease, particularly in young cats of up to 6 months of age. Ulcerative keratitis may accompany an herpes conjunctivitis, but usually only in the older cat. Antiviral agents such as idoxuridine (Kerecid, Allergan) and acyclovir (Zovirax, Wellcome) can prove valuable in the treatment of this condition. There is no adequate therapy for the treatment of reovirus and calicivirus infections. It is always sensible to

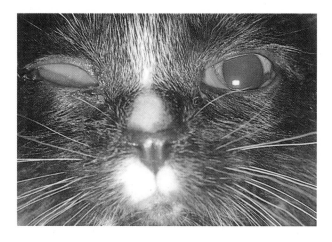

Fig. 9.8
Unilateral (right)
acute conjunctivitis
with chemosis.

check the FeLV and FIV state of the patients when viral infection is suspected.

Chlamydia psittaci is a significant cause of conjunctivitis in this species, and it may be accompanied by mild rhinitis. The organism is very sensitive to tetracycline therapy, but the disease can persist for months if left untreated. *Mycoplasma gatae* and *M. felis* can also cause conjunctivitis, but the disease is usually mild and self-limiting. Both organisms are sensitive to chloramphenicol.

Allergic conjunctivitis may be seasonal and accompanied by other indications of cause, while follicular conjunctivitis, a chronic disease characterized by the presence of enlarged lymphoid follicles on all the conjunctival surfaces, remains an aetiological mystery. It does not respond to any medical treatment but a cure may be obtained by the chemical cauterization of the follicles or their surgical removal.

Primary bacterial conjunctivitis appears to be an unusual entity but bacterial secondaries can complicate any conjunctivitis.

SYMBLEPHARON

Symblepharon is caused mainly by the chronic conjunctivitis usually associated with upper respiratory tract infections. Adhesions occur between the palpebral and the bulbar conjunctival tissues limiting eyelid movement, the membrana nictitans may be fixed in a protrused position while corneal symblepharon can render the eye blind if the area of adhesion is extensive. Keratoconjunctivitis sicca (Fig. 9.9) is similarly possible should the excretory ducts of the lacrimal gland be occluded.

Minor symblepharon is best left untreated but lagophthalmos must be relieved and corneal opacity can be reduced by superficial keratectomy and the subsequent prevention of readhesions.

MEMBRANA NICTITANS

Unilateral protrusion of the membrana nictitans is part of Horner's syndrome, accompanies trigeminal irritation or pain,

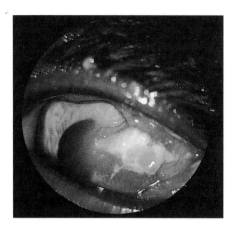

Fig. 9.9
Chronic "eosinophilic" keratoconjunctivitis
involving the dorsolateral limbus of the left eye.
Four-year-old DSH. The raised plaque of
heavily vascularized tissue covered by a
creamy-white "deposit" is seen involving both
the corneal and conjunctival tissues. (*Journal of
Small Animal Practice* (1982) 23, 85.)

may be due to symblepharon and may accompany proptosis due to orbital cellulitis or neoplasia. The aetiology of a bilateral protrusion should include these considerations but other factors such as systemic infection, malnutrition or any other form of systemic stress should be considered.

Retention of the membrana nictitans in its normal position is considered to be a function of the smooth muscle attached to the base of the structure. This muscle receives sympathetic innervation and postulated inflammatory disease of possible viral origin involving the peripheral sympathetic chain would result in loss of muscle tone and protrusion of the membrana nictitans (cf. Horner's syndrome in which ptosis, miosis and enophthalmos also accompany the protrusion of the membrana nictitans. The syndrome is due to a disruption of sympathetic nerve supply to the eye and its adnexa).

In this instance the protrusion is self limiting, usually lasting for approximately 8 weeks, and may be preceded by a gastroenteritis of short duration. Retraction of the protrused membranae nictitans can be obtained using topical 1% adrenaline (Eppy, SNP), or 2% phenylephrine (Minims, SNP), but such treatment can cause conjunctival irritation and is of cosmetic value only.

LACRIMAL SYSTEM

Acquired disease of the lacrimal system is due to inflammatory disease and the damage such processes may cause. Dacryoadenitis, inflammation of the lacrimal gland which can result in a keratoconjunctivitis sicca and dacryocystitis, inflammation of the lacrimal sac which can result in occlusion of the nasolacrimal duct, are difficult to identify as specific entities.

Keratoconjunctivitis sicca, dry eye, is most frequently associated with chronic conjunctivitis and adequate medical control is rarely possible when the Schirmer reading is low or zero. The frequent administration of a topical artificial tear preparation combined with the lacrimogenic effect of oral 1% pilocarpine represents the standard medical approach to this problem but parotid duct transposition is of proven value in terms of possible cure.

THE CORNEA

Acquired corneal disease is not uncommon in the cat. Laceration wounds that do not penetrate into the anterior chamber are treated simply, topical antibiosis being used prophylactically until re-epithelialization has been completed.

Small sealed penetration wounds without the inclusion of iridal tissue require treatment with topical and systemic antibiosis, and, in addition, corticosteroid and atropine therapy should be used to control any consequent uveitis. Extensive penetration wounds which have sealed without iris inclusion are similarly treated, but in addition a membrana flap can be used to cover the cornea during the healing period of approximately 14 days.

Long standing staphylomas (Fig. 9.10) are best left but in the management of the acute corneal wound in which there is iris inclusion, the extruded iridal material may be replaced into the anterior chamber, or removed should that prove impossible. The wound can then be sutured using 6/0 collagen and post-operative therapy must involve treatment of the attendant uveitis as well as antibiosis.

Keratitis in the cat is usually associated with conjunctivitis and both ulcerative and non-ulcerative forms are seen. Scrapings for culture and viral isolation are of distinct value in

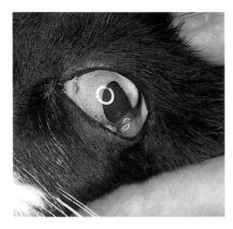

Fig. 9.10
Limbal staphyloma formation following corneal penetration. Left eye. Two-year-old DSH.

considering treatment. The membrana flap should be used in the treatment of superficial ulceration, whereas pedicle flaps constructed of bulbar conjunctiva offer a valuable approach to the management of the deep ulcer and the descemetocele. (Bistner *et al.*, 1977; Bedford, 1980).

Viral involvement in corneal disease must be considered as a differential diagnosis in patients presenting with both ulcerative and non-ulcerative keratitis and accompanying upper respiratory tract infection. The immunosuppressive effects of corticosteroid therapy can potentiate the infection but the use of idoxuridine can be most effective. The FeLV and FIV stati of the patient should be checked as routine.

A chronic granulomatous type of keratitis has been described in American cats as an eosinophilic or proliferative keratitis and an association with the eosinophilic granuloma complex has been suggested. A similar disease has recently been recorded in the United Kingdom (Bedford and Cotchin, 1983). Although the corneal lesion has the same gross appearance as the lesions described in America, differences have been seen in the histopathological picture and a marked conjunctival component is usually present. The disease is characterized by the presence of distinctive plaques of chronic inflammatory tissue on the corneal and adjacent conjunctival surfaces, the extent of the corneal lesion and the effect on vision varying considerably. Despite the bizarre appearance of this species-specific disease, it should not present a major problem to the practitioner for its incidence would appear to be low, the clinical features are diagnostically unique and both corrective and prophylactic therapy using megestrol acetate (Ovarid, Glaxo) are readily available.

The aetiology of a species-specific corneal necrosis or mummification remains unknown, but there is some indication that its incidence in the Persian and Siamese breed is somewhat greater than random selection would allow (Fig. 9.11) There is often a history of chronic ocular disease during which herpesvirus may have been isolated. The appearance of the lesion may be heralded by a brown staining of the central anterior stroma. This is gradually replaced by a well defined black plaque of tissue with a smooth or irregular surface that is usually raised above the level of the surrounding corneal epithelium. The condition may be accompanied by obvious discomfort, but many patients would appear to remain unaffected in this respect.

The stroma is involved to varying depths, even down to Descemet's membrane, and a surrounding zone of stromal inflammation is present. The disease may be bilateral but frequently affects only one cornea. With time the lesions will slough and this can represent an acceptable line of treatment when the patient remains comfortable. However keratectomy is advocated when the patient is in pain: removal of lesion together with some normal surrounding stroma is easily accomplished when the lesion is relatively superficial. However deep extension of the lesion will necessitate the use of a conjunctival pedicle graft or a corneal graft to effect successful

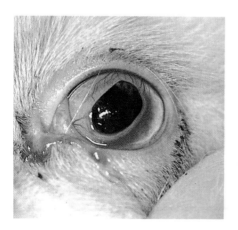

Fig. 9.11
Corneal necrosis. The classical black body appearance of the lesion. Left eye. Three-year-old Persian.

repair. Such surgery is not always successful, and the prognosis should be guarded.

Unlike the dog, corneal dystrophies are of extremely low incidence in the cat. Stromal oedema together with epithelial oedema and ulceration in association with stromal collagen and Descemet's membrane defects has been reported as an apparently recessively inherited disease in the Manx cat (Bistner *et al.*, 1976).

Lipid corneal degeneration may require treatment by superficial keratectomy if sight is impaired or there is additional corneal pathology.

THE UVEAL TRACT

Anterior uveitis is relatively common being related either to trauma or systemic disease. Corticosteroid and atropine therapy represent the standard approach to management. The specific cause may not always be defined, but feline leukaemia virus, toxoplasmosis and feline infectious peritonitis must always be considered in the differential diagnosis (Figs 9.12–9.14). The patient's FIV status should always be determined.

The diagnosis of toxoplasmosis is dependent upon the demonstration of a rapidly rising titre and the zoonotic aspect of the disease should be remembered when treatment is

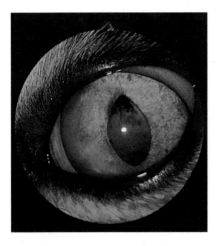

Fig. 9.12
Feline leukaemia. Neoplastic tissue change is seen involving the iris medial to the pupil. Left eye. Four-year-old DSH.

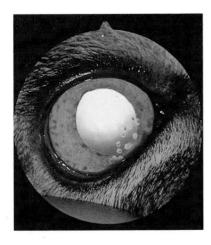

Fig. 9.13
Anterior uveitis in toxoplasmosis. Keratic
precipitates can be seen on the ventral corneal
mesothelium. Right eye. Two-year-old DSH.

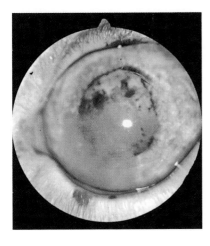

Fig. 9.14
Anterior uveitis in feline infectious peritonitis. The
iris is thickened, and the aterior chamber partially
filled with a fibrinous exudate. Left eye. Two-year-
old DSH.

attempted. The disease induces a low grade anterior uveitis
which may be characterized by the formation of keratic
precipitates or KPs, clumps of mononuclear inflammatory cells
adherent to the corneal mesothelium. A multifocal chorioretinitis may accompany the anterior uveitis and small bullous
retinal detachments can result.

In feline infectious peritonitis, the iris becomes thickened
and immobile and a marked fibrinoid exudate fills the anterior
chamber. Large clumps of exudate and inflammatory cells can

remain as sizeable structures attached to the anterior iris.

In early feline leukaemia low grade uveitis may be the only ocular feature apparent but later the iris becomes distorted by the presence of neoplastic tissue. The posterior uvea may also be involved and retinal detachments may occur.

The anterior uveal tract is the commonest site for intraocular neoplasia and of the primary tumours recorded in the cat, the malignant melanoma occurs most frequently (Fig. 9.15). Infiltration of the iridocorneal angle may cause secondary glaucoma and the liver and lungs are the common sites for metastases. Early enucleation represents the safest line of treatment, although metastasis is slow and both iridectomy and iridocyclectomy are possible when the tumour can be localized.

Adenocarcinoma of the ciliary epithelium is the next most common tumour either filling the retro-iridal space (Fig. 9.16) or extending into the anterior chamber through the peripheral iris. In addition, the uveal tract can be a site of carcinoma metastasis from the lungs, uterus and mammary gland.

One differential for the anterior uveal malignant melanoma is the anterior uveal (iris) cyst which may occur as the result of trauma, following uveitis or in old age. Cysts are only of clinical significance if they either impair vision or induce secondary glaucoma as the result of a pupillary block. Removal through a limbal section is easily achieved.

A second and unusual differential is iridal granuloma formation which may be part of the eosinophilic granuloma

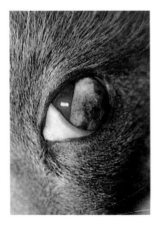

Fig. 9.15
Malignant melanoma of the ciliary body. The tumour has infiltrated the iris, and dark pigmentation is apparent in three areas. Malignant melanomas are highly vascular, and in this patient haemorrhage is clearly seen. Left eye. Seven-year-old DSH.

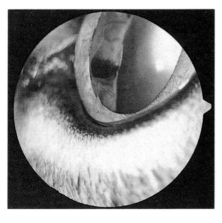

Fig. 9.16
Adenocarcinoma of the ciliary body filling the ventro-medial retro-iridal space. Left eye. Eight-year-old DSH.

complex. The author has seen this condition in two patients, and in both the lesion was responsive to megoestrol acetate therapy (Ovarid, Glaxo).

A syndrome characterized by persistent mydriasis not associated with amavrosis, mid-brain disease or trauma made an epidemic appearance in British cats several years ago (Nash *et al.*, 1982), but currently new cases are not occurring. It was commonly referred to as the Key–Gaskell syndrome. Various alimentary tract problems accompanied the mydriasis and the syndrome was attributed to an autonomic polyganglionopathy in which both sympathetic and parasympathetic ganglia demonstrated neurone loss. The aetiology remains unknown, but viral infection, unspecified toxicity and a possible nutritional involvement have all been examined.

Mydriasis, in association with peripapillary oedema, retinal neovascularization, ataxia and convulsions also occurs as the result of thiamine deficiency but vision remains unaffected.

THE LENS

Acquired disease of the feline lens occurs much less frequently than in its canine counterpart. Cataract is usually related to trauma, uveitis or senility and there is no evidence to suggest that the rare developmental cataract in the young cat is inherited.

The incidence of lens luxation (Fig. 9.17) is so low that any discussion of cause must remain incomplete. Dislocation can be associated with trauma or occur as the result of globe enlargement in glaucome (Fig. 9.18) but occasionally the cause may remain unknown.

Complete separation of the zonular attachments means that the lens can be displaced into the anterior chamber but the depth of this structure means that the lens can usually be accommodated without the risk of a pupillary block glaucoma.

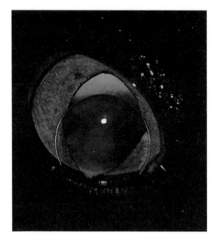

Fig. 9.17
Anterior lens luxation. Glaucoma is not present. Right eye. Five-year-old DSH.

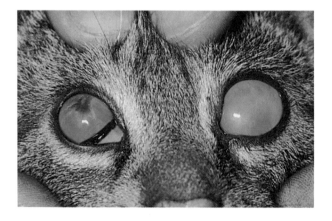

Fig. 9.18
Bilateral secondary glaucoma due to uveitis in 3-year-old DSH. Globe enlargement is most apparent in the left eye.

THE RETINA

Retinal disease may occur as a primary defect or may be related to other concurrent ocular or systemic disease. In the latter instance diagnosis may be difficult if extensive anterior segment changes are present.

Retinitis and chorioretinitis occur in association with toxoplasmosis, feline leukaemia and feline infectious peritonitis, and routine examination should include the FIV status of the patient. Intraretinal and preretinal haemorrhages may be seen in anaemia and thrombocytopaenia.

Retinal detachment is due to a posterior uveitis, hypertension or neoplasia. Intraretinal glycolipid buildup has been seen in cats with GM_2 gangliosidosis.

In lipaemia retinalis the superficial retinal blood vessels in the nontapetal fundus (Fig. 9.19) appear yellow or orange in colour, this anomaly being related to hyperlipidaemia which may be corrected by the appropriate attention to diet.

The aetiology of retinal degeneration involves both nutritional and hereditary considerations. A recessively inherited rod/cone dysplasia has been recorded in a litter of Persian kittens (Rubin and Lipton, 1973), while a dominantly inherited rod/cone dysplasia has been described in a closed colony of Abyssinian cats (Barnett and Curtis, 1985). In Sweden a bilateral generalized retinal degeneration first appearing at 12–13 months of age has been described for this latter

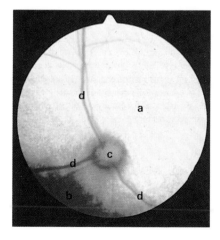

Fig. 9.19
The normal feline fundus. Right eye. Two-year-old DSH. a, Tapetal fundus; b, non-tapetal fundus; c, optic disc (optic papilla); d, superficial retinal vasculature.

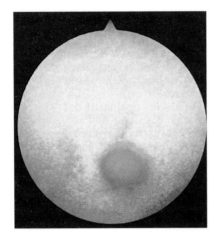

Fig. 9.20
Generalized retinal atrophy in a 10-year-old
Siamese. Right eye.

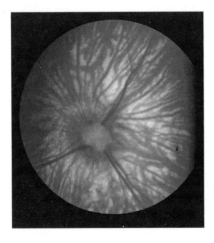

Fig. 9.21
The fundus of a 12 month-old blue eyed white DSH
cat. There is no tapetum and the lack of both
retinal and choroidal pigmentation highlights the
choroidal vasculature against the white background
of the sclera.

breed, the disease being inherited as a simple recessive trait
(Narfstrom and Nilsson, 1983). In the UK, generalized retinal
degeneration occurs in middle-aged and older cats, but the
aetiology remains unknown. The Siamese and, again, the
Abyssinian have been involved, but the disease is also seen
in less exotic individuals (Fig. 9.20). Early stages of this disease
are rarely seen, most patients being presented with extensive
neuroretinal degeneration as witnessed by a loss of pupillary
light reflex, mydriasis, increased tapetal reflectivity and retinal

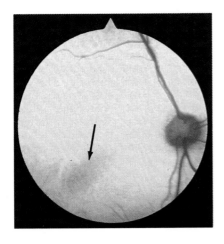

Fig. 9.22
FCRD in a 16'year-old Siamese. Right eye.

blood vessel attenuation (Fig. 9.21). It has been postulated that one possible cause is long-term deficiency of the essential aminosulphonic acid taurine. As a species, the cat cannot synthesize taurine to any useful extent, and dietary deficiency is seen as a cardiomyopathy or retinal degeneration. The initial retinal lesion is a focal central zone of degeneration involving the area centralis (Barnett and Burger, 1980), a clinical picture which was described as FCRD (feline central retinal degeneration) by earlier workers (Bellhorn and Fischer, 1970) (Fig. 9.22). The lesion may extend linearly to involve the nasal portion of the tapetal fundus and extensive neuroretinal degeneration may accompany long-term deprivation. Taurine deficiency may be related to its impaired metabolism as well as dietary insufficiency, and the bioavailability of taurine in this species is a subject of current research. The possible inheritance of generalized retinal degeneration in the older cat has yet to be substantiated, but it too is currently being investigated.

GLAUCOMA

Glaucoma is uncommon in cats and is usually present as a secondary disease process to trauma, uveitis and intraocular neoplasia. A primary open angle type of chronic glaucoma does occur and is characterized by gradual globe enlargement,

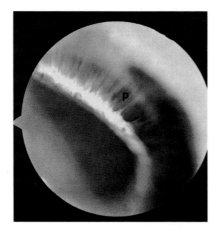

Fig. 9.23
A goniophotograph of the open drainage angle in a
5 year old DSH presenting with chronic glaucoma.
The pectinate fibres (P) can be clearly
distinguished spanning the entrance to the ciliary
cleft.

secondary lens luxation and progressive loss of vision (Fig. 9.23).

The iridocorneal (drainage) angle remains open and dichlor-phenamide (Daranide; Merck, Sharpe and Dohme) therapy can be effective, although potassium depletion is always a possible complication.

For other types of glaucoma, treatment is best achieved by surgery, the technique of corneoscleral trephination with peripheral iridectomy offering a reasonable approach to the problem (Bedford, 1977).

REFERENCES

Barnett, K. C. & Burger, I. H. (1980). *Journal of Small Animal Practice* **21**, 52.
Barnett, K. C. & Curtis, R. (1988). *Journal of Heredity* **76**, 168.
Bedford, P. G. C. (1977). *Journal of Small Animal Practice* **18**, 713.
Bedford, P. G. C. (1980). *In Practice* **2**, 5.
Bedford, P. G. C. & Cotchin, E. (1983). *Journal of Small Animal Practice* **23**, 85.
Bellhorn, R. W. & Fischer, C. A. (1970). *Journal of the American Veterinary Medical Association* **157**, 842.
Bistner, S. I., Aguirre, G. & Shively, J. N. (1976). *Ophthalmology* **15**, 15.
Bistner, S. I., Aguirre, G. & Batik, G. (1977). *Atlas of Veterinary Ophthalmic Surgery*. W. B. Saunders, Philadelphia.
Harvey, C. E. (1977). Exploration of the orbit. In *Atlas of Veterinary Ophthalmic*

Surgery (eds S. I. Bistner, G. Aguirre & G. Batik). W. B. Saunders, Philadelphia.

Narfstrom, K. & Nilsson, S. E. G. (1983). *Veterinary Record* **112**, 525.

Nash, A. S., Griffiths, I. R. & Sharp, J. N. H. (1982). *Veterinary Record* **25**, 307.

Peiffer, R. L. (1981) Feline ophthalmology. In *Veterinary Ophthalmology* (ed. K. N. Gelatt). Lea and Febiger, Philadelphia.

Rubin, L. F. & Lipton, D. E. (1973). *Journal of the American Veterinary Medical Association* **162**, 467.

CHAPTER 10

Skin Diseases

KEITH THODAY

INTRODUCTION

Skin diseases may be classified according to aetiology into two basic categories, those factors acting on the skin from within the animal (the internal factors) and those acting on it from the environment (the external factors) (Fig. 10.1). However, certain diseases, such as allergy, and certain types of neoplasia may require an interaction of both an internal predisposition and an external stimulus prior to developing the condition. There are also many conditions which, at present, must be classified as idiopathic.

INTERNAL FACTORS

GENETIC OR CONGENITAL

A number of conditions which have a genetic or congenital basis have been recorded in the cat. All are rare and, while of considerable interest to the dermatologist, are of minimal importance to the practitioner.

In all of these conditions, owners should be strongly persuaded not to use affected animals for breeding.

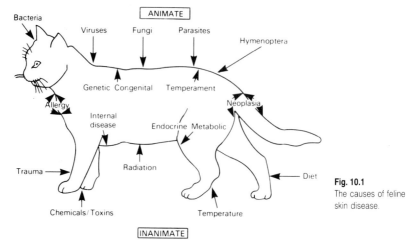

Fig. 10.1
The causes of feline skin disease.

Alopecia universalis

Affected cats are totally alopecic except for whiskers. The skin is oily and may be traumatized by the cat when cleaning.

Hereditary hypotrichosis

Hereditary hypotrichosis has been recorded in the Siamese and the Devon Rex breeds (Fig. 10.2).

Cutaneous asthenia

Cutaneous asthenia (Ehlers–Danlos syndrome, dermato-sparaxis) is a rare group of diseases which may be characterized by skin hyperextensibility and fragility and by tearing following minimal trauma.

The Chediak–Higashi syndrome

The Chediak–Higashi syndrome (oculocutaneous albinism) is a recently described condition seen in blue-smoke, yellow-eyed, Persian cats characterized clinically by partial albinism of the eyes and haircoat, an increased susceptibility to infection and a bleeding tendency.

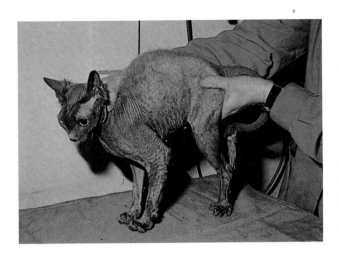

Fig. 10.2
Hereditary
hypotrichosis in a
female Devon rex
cat. A number of
kittens born to it were
also affected.

TEMPERAMENT

Individual response

Individual variation in response to cutaneous insults markedly affects presenting signs. In some animals a mild degree of pruritus may be unbearable and result in severe self-inflicted injury, whereas in more stoical individuals severe sensory stimuli may be tolerated with minimal self-mutilation.

Neurodermatitis

A condition characterized by excessive licking, seen primarily in "highly strung" breeds (Siamese, Abyssinian and Burmese) is reported to be an anxiety neurosis and has been termed "neurodermatitis". There appears to be considerable doubt as to the validity of this diagnosis in many cases to which it has been ascribed.

Muller and Kirk (1976) reported that the primary or initiating cause may be a dermatitis with pruritus, infected ears or anal sacs which would make a diagnosis of neurodermatitis seem dubious. In other cases, the precipitating factor is a change in the cat's life-cycle (e.g. new home, new baby or pet, etc.) which is said to result in the lesions in a basically neurotic individual.

Lesions are variable but usually occur in areas the cat can lick easily, such as the dorsal lumbo-sacral area, tail, medial thighs and ventral abdomen. An erythematous patch or streak, or an area of partial alopecia with broken hairs, is seen. In Siamese cats, hairs may regrow a darker colour.

Diagnosis is based on elimination of physical causes, such as fleas, *Cheyletiella* spp. infestation, aberrant *Otodectes* spp. infestation, anal sac impaction, foreign bodies, previous bone injury and neurological disease. Improvement on glucocorticoid therapy may help to rule out a diagnosis of neurodermatitis.

Treatment should be directed at determining and removing, where possible, the cause of anxiety. Oral diazepam or phenobarbitone may be required in the short or long term and megoestrol acetate is also reported to be effective.

ENDOCRINE/METABOLIC FACTORS

Feline endocrine alopecia

The aetiology of feline endocrine alopecia (Fig. 10.3) is unknown but is presumed to be hormonal deficiency or imbalance because it usually responds well to various hormonal therapies. The condition affects adult males and females at varying intervals after neutering. Occasionally, entire cats are affected and it is uncommon in purebred cats.

The condition is bilaterally symmetrical and usually begins over the perineal and genital regions, the posterior and medial thighs or the ventral abdomen. The forelegs (elbow to carpus) are frequently affected. In long-standing cases, hair is lost over the ventral two-thirds of the lateral abdomen and, less commonly, the thorax. There is diffuse alopecia, with particular loss of primary hairs. In most cases, the skin is otherwise macroscopically normal with no pruritus. Occasionally there may be areas of erythema and pruritus resulting in fracture of hairs.

Diagnosis is presently based on history and physical examination. However, other conditions may show a similar clinical appearance. Cases of apparent endocrine alopecia often show evidence of fleas on detailed examination and/or respond to treatment with a parasiticide alone. True endocrine alopecia will respond, variably, to various therapeutic regimes such as oral thyroid hormones, megoestrol acetate and oral, depot injectable or implanted testosterone. Continuous low dose or intermittent high dose therapy is usually required to maintain normality.

Hypothyroidism

Naturally occurring feline hypothyroidism has not, as yet, been satisfactorily confirmed.

Hyperadrenocorticalism

Naturally occurring hyperadrenocoriticalism is very rare in cats. Iatrogenic cases resulting from the long-term adminis-tration of glucocorticoids, usually in the control of undiagnosed pruritus, are not as uncommon as the paucity of literature on the subject would suggest. Clinical signs of polyuria, polydipsia, polyphagia and pendulous abdomen due to hepa-tomegaly and thinning of the abdominal musculature (but without the classical skin changes seen in the condition in the dog) have been seen. The condition responds completely to gradual reduction and cessation of glucocorticoid therapy.

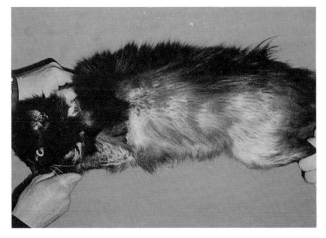

Fig. 10.3
Feline endocrine
alopecia.

INTERNAL DISEASE

The skin is an excellent indicator of general health and a large number of internal diseases may, therefore, result in cutaneous lesions. Some are of particular note.

In each case, the diagnosis is suggested by the history and physical examination and confirmed by standard laboratory tests.

Renal disease

In end-stage kidney disease, seborrhoea sicca (Fig. 10.4) is common and there may be a diffuse alopecia, with or without low-grade pruritus.

Hepatic disease

Hepatic disease may result in diffuse alopecia and pruritus. The skin is dry, often with bran-like scales, particularly over the trunk.

Diabetes mellitus

This commonly results in a dry haircoat and seborrhoea sicca, with or without mild pruritus.

Maldigestion or malabsorption diseases

These may result in fatty acid deficiency with resultant dry or greasy seborrhoea which is sometimes pruritic.

EXTERNAL FACTORS

ANIMATE

Bacteria

With the exception of cellulitis and abscesses, usually resulting from bites and scratches, bacterial skin diseases of the cat are uncommon.

Cellulitis and abscess

Cellulitis and abscesses are most frequent in entire males but entire females and neuters may be affected. The limbs, tail, head and face are the most common sites. The primary lesion is one or more pairs of puncture wounds. The course of the disease is variable, depending to a great extent on the site, cellulitis being most common in areas where dead space is minimal. The skin is inflamed, swollen and tender or painful. Systemic signs vary from absent to severe (anorexia, pyrexia, depression).

The organism most commonly isolated in *Pasteurella multocida* but β-haemolytic streptococci and *Fusiformis* species are

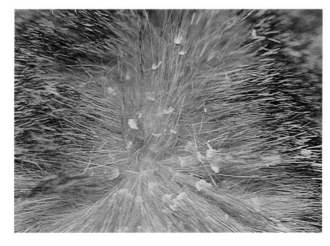

Fig. 10.4
Seborrhoea sicca in a cat with longstanding hepatic disease.

also regularly isolated. All are found as part of the cat's normal oral flora.

Infections as a sequel to cat bites are so frequent that prophylactic antibiosis using oral or parenteral penicillins is always justified if the lesion can be positively identified. Cellulitis should be fomented and treated similarly but discrete abscesses should merely be encouraged to develop by hot fomentations and allowed to burst or be lanced. Drainage should be promoted by cleaning and by mechanically opening the sinus twice daily (e.g. by using the nozzle of an empty antibiotic tube) until pus production ceases.

Myobacteria

Feline cutaneous tuberculosis, resulting from infection with *Mycobacterium bovis* and, less commonly, *M. tuberculosis* is now of minimal importance due to control of the diseases in both cattle and man. Lesions are single or multiple plaques, nodules and ulcers. Diagnosis relies on the finding of acid-fast bacilli in open lesions, culture and skin biopsy. After a positive diagnosis, the public health authorities should be notified and the cat euthanased.

Infections with other (non-tubercular) mycobacteria, including *M. lepraemurium, M. ulcerans, M. fortuitum* and *M. xenopi* have been recorded rarely. The lesions are usually single or multiple, non-painful, cutaneous or subcutaneous nodules or abscesses, frequently occurring over the head and limbs. They do not spread but enlarge slowly. Diagnosis is by direct smears from open lesions, culture and skin biopsy. Surgery is the treatment of choice, where feasible. Medical therapy is less reliable but successes have been reported using dapsone, tetracycline and chloramphenicol.

Actinomycetes

Cutaneous infections with *Actinomyces* and *Nocardia* species have been observed rarely in cats. Both infections are characterized by the formation of single or multiple, painful, pyogranulomatous abscesses discharging pus containing mycelial clumps ("sulphur granules"), sometimes with blood, via drainage tracts. Lesions may ulcerate and apparently heal, to be followed by local recurrence. The diagnosis is confirmed by demonstrating the organisms in direct smears of exudate after crushing the mycelial clumps, culture and biopsy. Treatment should combine prolonged high-level systemic or oral antibiosis (penicillin, sulphadiazine, trimethoprim/sulphadiazine combination) with twice-daily lavage of the tracts using saline or diluted 20 volumes hydrogen peroxide, followed by flushing of the tracts with the appropriate antibiotic. Oral potassium iodide (30–150 mg daily in dilute solution) has effective proteolytic actions, thinning discharges, increasing drainage and removing remaining foci of infection. Concentrated solutions may result in gastric irritation and should not be used.

Viruses

Until recently, cutaneous lesions due to viral infections were not recognized in cats. A number of viruses, however, have now been identified in association with skin disease, although a causal relationship is not proven for all.

It is likely that as virus isolation becomes commercially more available, the role of such agents in feline dermatoses will become better defined.

Feline leukaemia virus

Skin conditions which have been seen in feline leukaemia virus-positive cats include generalized seborrhoea, eosinophilic (rodent) ulcers and various forms of neoplasia (cutaneous lymphosarcoma, fibrosarcoma and liposarcoma). In addition, long-standing or recurrent infections and poor wound healing may result from the immunosuppressive actions of the virus. Such infections are reported to respond more satisfactorily to an antibiotic/glucocorticoid combination then to antibiotics alone. It is prudent to investigate the leukaemia virus status of cats presented with such diseases.

Picornavirus

A picornavirus, feline calicivirus, has been isolated from vesicles, erosions and ulcers on the feet and in the oral cavity of a young cat. The lesions cleared with symptomatic therapy. Virus particles suggestive of a picornavirus (calicivirus) have also been observed in biopsies from a cat with eosinophilic granuloma complex. A causal relationship was not, however, implied.

Feline herpesvirus (feline viral rhinotracheitis)

Feline herpesvirus has been isolated from skin ulcers in cats but it is not clear whether the virus was the primary cause of the lesions in all cases.

Cowpox

Cowpox virus was isolated from alopecic, ulcerated, nodular skin lesions in a cat which also had dyspnoea in association with a pleural effusion.

Fungi

Superficial infections (dermatomycosis)

Dermatophytes are fungi that invade only the dead, keratinized layers of the skin and its adnexa – the stratum corneum, the hair above the matrix cells and, occasionally, the nails. Infection is via direct contact with an infected animal or indirectly by contact with desquamated material free in the environment or on fomites such as combs or brushes. Airborne transmission between cats has been demonstrated. Material may remain viable in the environment for long periods. All ages and breeds of animal are susceptible to infection but a number of predisposing factors are known to exist (Table 10.1).

Although 14 species of dermatophyte have been isolated from cats, 98% of cases in the United Kingdom are caused by *Microsporum canis*.

On exposure to a dermatophyte, the organism may or may not establish residence. Even if it does, clinical signs may not be produced. Lesions are common over the head and legs but large areas of the trunk may be affected. The classical "ringworm" lesion (Fig. 10.5) is a rapidly growing, circular patch of partial or total alopecia surrounding or containing broken hairs. The skin is dry and usually covered with greyish scale, but may be erythematous. Other manifestations include small or large, irregularly shaped, diffuse lesions with similar skin changes to those above; localized or generalized papular dermatitis with skin crusting, with or without marked alopecia and secondary bacterial infection, and localized or generalized seborrhoea sicca.

Pruritus is unusual and more commonly associated with infection with *Trichophyton* species (Fig. 10.6) or secondary bacterial involvement. On rare occasions, firm or soft, painful or pruritic nodules are seen which may ulcerate and develop draining tracts (kerion formation).

The fine, long-haired breeds, such as the Persian, may be almost symptomless carriers of *M. canis*. Such cases are potentially very important in the spread of the disease in catteries and the home. *M. canis* is commonly transmitted to man and affected owners should be advised to consult their medical practitioners.

Table 10.1 Factors predisposing to dermatophyte infections.

Age – young animals predisposed (low skin fatty acid concentration, lack of acquired immunity)

Lack of acquired resistance

Defective cell-mediated immunity

Skin defects – broken skin probably required for establishment of initial infection

Nutritional deficiencies – in particular protein and Vitamin A

Existing systemic illness

Climate – high temperature, high humidity

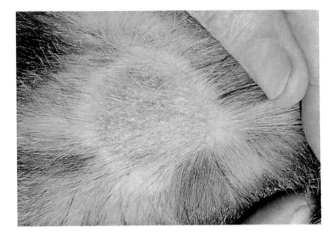

Fig. 10.5
The textbook
"ringworm" lesion:
Microsporum canis.
(Courtesy C. P.
Mackenzie.)

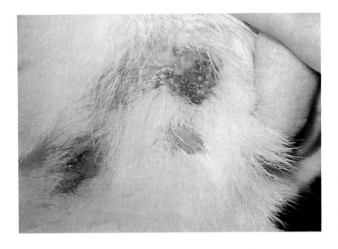

Fig. 10.6
*Tricophyton
mentagrophytes*
infection, dorsal
neck.

The laboratory procedures for the diagnosis of dermato-mycosis are technically simple but require experience in their interpretation to avoid false positive results. Animals should initially be examined with ultraviolet (Wood's) light. Approximately 60% of strains of *M. canis* fluoresce. *M. audouni, M. distortum, M. incurvata* and also *Tricophyton quinckeanum* may show a response. The positive apple-green fluorescence of affected hairs must be distinguished from the bluish appearance of dust and from the irridescence or true fluorescence of some topical applications. Fluorescence is not shown by skin scales, crusts or laboratory fungal cultures.

Material should then be collected for microscopic examination and culture. With lesions that fluoresce, affected hairs should be chosen but otherwise damaged hairs should be plucked with epilation forceps, not cut, and the scales and crusts removed with a blunt scalpel blade. Part of the material should be examined by direct microscopy after warming gently in 10% potassium hydroxide solution. Material may also be stained using lactophenol cotton blue or blue-black ink. Fungal arthrospores are observed as small, spherical, refractile bodies which, with *Microsporum* species, frequently obliterate the anatomical features of the hair.

The remainder of the sample should be inoculated on to a suitable medium (e.g. Sabouraud's or mycobiotic agar) and cultured at room temperature. Alternatively, a suitable inoculum may be collected by brushing the coat with a sterile toothbrush. However, fungal growth does not confirm the presence of a pathogen as contaminants are common. The morphology of the colony, the colour changes produced during its growth and the microscopic appearance of the macroconidia in wet preparations are diagnostic of the causal organism.

Dermatomycosis is commonly a self-limiting disease but it should be treated in every case. Prior to drug therapy, potentially infected keratin should be removed by close clipping. Because diffuse infection is common in cats, even those superficially showing only small numbers of lesions, should have total body clips. This seemingly time-consuming and costly procedure is, in fact, time-saving and economically viable because it reduces the duration of treatment. Clippings should be disposed of carefully, preferably by burning.

The fungistatic antibiotic, griseofulvin, should be used in all cases. Fat enhances its absorption, 2–5 ml of corn oil being effective and readily taken by cats. The drug is teratogenic and is therefore contra-indicated in pregnancy. The animal should be re-examined at the end of 1 month and re-clipped but treatment should be continued until the animal is clinically free of symptoms and cultures are negative.

Topical therapy with certain preparations is impractical and expensive and the lack of patient cooperation and dense body hair causes problems during and after application.

In-contact animals should be examined for evidence of

infection and, if negative, treated with griseofulvin at full
therapeutic dosage for 2 weeks.

Fungal spores may remain viable in shed material for at
least 7 months and possibly as long as 7 years, and it is
important to attempt to reduce environmental contamination.
In the home environment, vacuum cleaning, disposal of
bedding and other possibly infected equipment would be
most effective. In catteries, recommended disinfectants include
iodine, formalin, alcohol, chlorhexidine, sodium hypochlorite
and steam.

The elimination of fungal infections from cat colonies is a
specialized undertaking, requiring application and persistence
on the part of both owner and veterinary surgeon. A possible
approach has been documented by Dawson and Noddle (1968).

Intermediate and deep mycoses

Intermediate mycoses are so called because causal organisms
usually affect the skin and mucosae but occasionally become
deeper, whereas deep mycoses are systemic infections with
possible secondary cutaneous lesions. Both manifestations of
fungal disease have been recognized but are very rare in cats
in the United Kingdom.

Parasites

Parasitic infestations are the single most important cause of
feline skin disease (Table 10.2). A number are also potentially
transmissible to man, causing troublesome eruptions which
may defy medical diagnosis in the absence of examination of
the affected pet.

Ticks

Ticks are not host-specific but have host preferences and these
extend to the cat only infrequently. While discomfort may be
seen at the site of attachment and pruritus has been reported
in severe infestations, cats usually tolerate ticks well and they
are presented by concerned owners who have suddenly

Table 10.2 Important causes of parasitic dermatoses of the cat in the UK. (Where a number of genera may be involved, the most common are given in parentheses.)

Ticks	– Various (*Ixodes hexagonus*)
Fleas	– Various (*Ctenocephalides felis, Spilopsyllus cuniculi, Archaeopsyllus erinacei*)
Lice	– *Felicola subrostratus*
Mites	– *Otodectes cynotis* Cheyletiella (*Cheyletiella blakei*) *Trombicula autumnalis*
Flies	– Various

noticed a "growth or cyst". Any area of the body may be affected but the head, neck and limbs are most commonly involved.

Ticks may be removed manually by grasping the capitulum as close as possible to the skin using forceps and pulling gently in a straight line. Care must be taken to ensure that the mouthparts are completely removed or a foreign-body granuloma may develop. Occasionally such reactions occur in the absence of retained mouthparts, suggesting a chronic immunological reaction (perhaps due to arthropod antigens bound to dermal collagen) which can often be aborted by intralesional glucocorticoids. After, or in place of, manual removal, the animal should be treated with a reliable parasiticide to remove any parasites remaining in the coat.

Fleas

Fleas are the most important parasitic cause of skin disease in the cat. In the UK, the species most commonly found on cats are *Ctenocephalides felis* (94%), *Spilopsyllus cuniculi* (4%) and *Archaeopsyllus erinacei* (1%). They are facultative parasites, much of the life-cycle being spent away from the host in carpets, furnishings, baskets or the corners of rooms.

The clinical signs of infestation vary between individuals, the marked signs in some being due to irritant reactions or hypersensitivity to components of flea saliva. The allergens are haptens requiring conjugation with a dermal component, probably collagen, prior to becoming antigenic. The allergic reaction may involve either delayed (cell-mediated) or immediate (antibody-mediated) responses or, more commonly, a combination of the two. Fleas may be found on any age of animal but allergic reactions are rare in the young.

In non-sensitized individuals, response to bites is minimal and results in mild pruritus and excoriation. In allergic individuals, pruritus is marked over the predilection sites – the dorsal lumbosacral area, the ventral abdomen, the medial aspects of the hindlegs and sometimes the neck. The lesions, known as miliary dermatitis, are small papules topped by hard, dry, brown exudate. Self-inflicted injury causes the hair shaft to break near the skin causing diffuse alopecia and, occasionally, areas of acute moist dermatitis.

Diagnosis is by identification of the parasite or its brown or black, comma-shaped faeces which form a reddish-brown halo around them on moist cotton wool.

Treatment should be directed at ridding both the animal and its immediate environment of the parasite and at preventing, or at least minimizing, re-infestation. Affected and in-contact animals should be sprayed or dusted with an effective parasiticide, e.g. dichlorvos-fenitrothion combination or pyrethrum. Regular prophylactic treatment may be required, particularly in the case of hypersensitivity. Short-term glucocorticoids or megoestrol acetate may be required occasionally to reduce pruritus and self-inflicted injury.

To break the life-cycle, the whole environment should be vacuum cleaned at one time, the contents of the dust-bag being burned. Parasiticidal treatment of the environment using, for example, iodofenphos and dichlorvos may be helpful in severe infestations.

Lice

The biting louse *Felicola subrostratus* is occasionally seen on cats. Infestation produces few direct lesions but results in pruritus and, therefore, self-inflicted injury.

Lice are obligatory parasites reproducing on the host and cementing their eggs to hairs. Identification of the parasite or its "nits" confirms the diagnosis. Thorough treatment with almost any parasiticide usually results in rapid clearing of the condition.

Otodectes

The ear mite, *Otodectes cynotis*, is a relatively large, surface-living, obligatory parasite. While principally inhabiting the ear, it may be found on other areas of the body, particularly the head, interscapular area and tail. The parasite is highly contagious and is commonly transferred to dogs.

A thick, waxy, reddish-brown discharge is produced as a result of the mites' activities and this forms a protective layer around them. The degree of irritation varies markedly between individuals. In some, it is minimal but, in others, it may be intense and is manifested by head-shaking and scratching with the hind-feet, producing excoriation of the pinnae and, occasionally, haematoma formation. Subsequent infection of the ear canal by bacteria and yeasts may result.

Diagnosis is by auroscopic inspection or microscopic observation of the mite after warming exudate with 10% potassium hydroxide. Treatment of uncomplicated otodectic otitis should be with a simple parasiticidal preparation instilled into the external ear canal. All in-contact cats and dogs should be dealt with similarly because of the problems of contagion. As the parasite may be found elsewhere on the body, persistent or recurrent cases should, in addition, be treated with a general parasiticide such as dichlorvos/fenitrothion combination or pyrethrum. Where bacterial infection exists, antibiotic therapy is indicated, in most cases topical treatment alone being effective.

Cheyletiella

Cheyletiella species are surface-living mites just visible to the naked eye. The entire life-cycle (34 days) takes place on the host and eggs are attached to hairs. However, mites may live off the body for up to 10 days. Three species have been reported as infesting cats – *C. blakei* (the usual cat species), *C. parasitivorax* (usually found on rabbits) and *C. yasguri* (usually found on dogs).

There is no apparent breed, sex or age predisposition. The predilection site is the dorsum but response to infestation is variable. Pruritus may be absent or severe. Clinical signs include mild to moderate, dry, dorsal scaling, miliary dermatitis, pruritus without skin changes or a carrier state. Lesions in the owners are extremely common, even in the absence of signs in the cat, but resolve gradually once the infested animal has been treated.

Diagnosis may be made by direct inspection of the skin, with or without a magnifying lens and by microscopic examination of coat brushings or superficial skin scrapings. Infestation is frequently resistant to treatment with parasiticides in powder or aerosol form because the pseudo-tunnels produced by the mites in dermal debris prevent contact with the agent. One per cent selenium sulphide or sulphur washes are very effective and should be repeated three times at weekly intervals. In-contact dogs, cats and rabbits should be examined and treated similarly.

Trombicula autumnalis

Seasonal infestation with larvae of the harvest mite, *Trombicula autumnalis*, produces variable reactions in the skin of cats. The infestation is obtained from grass and the feet and head (particularly the ears) are commonly affected. Variable degrees of hyperaemia, papular dermatitis, pruritus and resultant self-excoriation and alopecia are produced.

The diagnosis is usually suspected because of the seasonal (late summer and autumn) nature of the disease and the distribution pattern. It is confirmed by identifying the 0.2 mm long, orange to red larvae either macro- or microscopically. Treatment with one application of any reliable, suitable parasiticide (e.g. dichlorvos/fenitrothion sprays, pyrethrum powder, selenium sulphide or sulphur washes) suffices because the adults are not parasitic and do not breed on the cat. Rarely, short-term glucocorticoids may be required to control severe pruritus.

Notoedres

Notoedric mange (feline scabies) is an intensely irritating, highly contagious, scaling dermatosis caused by infestation with the burrowing microscopic parasite, *Notoedres cati*. The mite is an obligatory parasite, surviving for only a few days off the host. The disease is now very rare in the UK and, in recent years, outbreaks have been confined largely to wild cat colonies.

Classically, the lesions begin on the borders of the ears and quickly spread to the upper surfaces, the face, neck, elbows and feet. The skin becomes thickened, covered with crusts and intense pruritus soon leads to self-inflicted injury with alopecia and secondary infection. Intensely pruritic papules may be present in the owners of affected animals. Diagnosis may be confirmed by the demonstration of the mite in deep skin scrapings.

Prior to parasiticidal treatment, the crusts should be softened with liquid paraffin or medicated soap solution. Preparations such as 1% selenium sulphide or sulphur baths are the treatment of choice because of their combined parasiticidal and anti-seborrhoeic activity. Treatment should be given at weekly intervals for 4–6 weeks. In-contact cats, dogs and rabbits should be treated similarly. Where necessary, short-term glucocorticoids are helpful in controlling pruritus.

Demodex

Demodicosis is a very rare disease of the cat due to the parasite *Demodex cati*. Little information is available about this parasite but details of the pathogenesis of the disease are assumed to be similar to the canine condition. Both local and generalized forms have been reported.

Myiasis

Cutaneous myiasis is an uncommon disease of cats affecting principally sick or injured animals. Blowflies and fresh flies lay their eggs on areas of coat covered in urine, faeces, discharges (commonly the perineum, genitals or eyes) or in

open wounds. The resultant larvae produce enzymes which
cause painful ulcers that may coalesce. Undermining is common and a foul, putrid odour is present.

Initially, the lesions should be clipped and cleaned with
antiseptic soap solution. The larvae should then be manually
removed or flushed out and a topical antibiotic suspension
applied. The coat, but not the lesions, should be treated with
a suitable parasiticide and efforts made to determine the cause
of the debility.

Hymenoptera

Bee and wasp stings are occasionally seen during the summer
months, particularly in the early or late part of the season
when the insects are torpid. Young, lively and inquisitive
animals are most commonly affected, usually on the face or
feet. Pain is followed by local oedema and hyperaemia of the
affected area. When a sting has been injected, it should first
be removed and, where feasible, cold compresses applied.
Antihistamines may be of limited value. Glucocorticoids may
be required in severe cases and are always indicated when
the lesion is in the oral cavity because the resultant oedema
may cause airway obstruction.

INANIMATE

Trauma

The skin forms a protective surface between the internal and
external environments and physical damage is a natural
hazard. Contusions, abrasions and lacerations are regularly
seen from a variety of causes and require little discussion
here. Physical irritant contact dermatitis on the feet, due to
agents such as sand and gravel, is uncommon in cats.

Chemicals and toxins

Chemical irritant contact dermatitis

Chemical irritant dermatitis is uncommon in cats and may
result from the application of primary irritants or so-called

relative primary irritants (Fig. 10.7). The latter are corrosive agents in low concentration or substances of low potency (e.g. soap, detergents, disinfectants and solvents) which, in certain individuals, on repeated application may produce irritation, inflammation and pruritus.

Unless the irritant is a liquid, hairy skin is not affected, lesions affecting the relatively glabrous ventral surfaces (chin, axillae, abdomen, feet) and the inner aspects of the pinnae, the medial thighs and perineum. Lesions vary from mild erythema to dramatic necrosis depending on the nature of the agent. Secondary infections occur rapidly.

Diagnosis is by history, physical signs and provocative exposure, if necessary. Treatment involves cleaning of the skin, using "universal" solvents, if necessary. Such treatment must be extremely thorough, otherwise the cat will attempt to complete the task with potentially disastrous results. Topical and systemic glucocorticoids and antibiotics may be required together with future avoidance of the irritant.

Chemical irritant dermatitis due to the organophosphorus compound dichlorovos and, occasionally, to carbamates has been reported in cats as a result of wearing flea-collars. The author has recognized flea collar dermatitis on only one occasion and agrees with Scott (1989) who wrote "Experiences and studies cause me to believe that flea-collar dermatitis and other flea-collar related disorders are, in general, only slightly more common than hen's teeth".

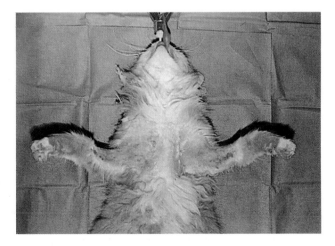

Fig. 10.7
Chemical irritant dermatitis. Turpentine substitute was used by the owner to remove paint from the coat.

Thallium poisoning

Thallium is a cumulative general cell poison, originally used as a rodenticide which may result in cutaneous signs of alopecia, erythema and necrosis of the skin. Its sale is now illegal in the UK.

Radiation

Feline solar dermatitis (Fig. 10.8) is a chronic inflammation of the pinna tips and, occasionally, of the eyelids and nasal skin of white or partially white cats supposedly due to the ultraviolet wavelengths of sunlight. Blue-eyed cats are said to be more commonly affected. While being more common in sunny districts other factors may be involved in the aetiology (e.g. specific genetic predisposition, hypersensitivity to sunlight, photosensitive pigments, etc.).

Early changes may be seen in young cats and tend to increase in severity each year. The skin of the ear tips initially show signs of severe sunburn with hyperaemia, scale, crust and pain. The resultant damage to hair follicles causes further thinning to the hair covering, making the pinna more susceptible to injury. In the early stages the lesions heal during the colder months but, as it progresses, the cartilage is damaged causing the pinnae to curl up at the edges. Eventually, an ulcerating, squamous cell carcinoma may be produced. Diagnosis is by physical examination and biopsy, if necessary.

The aim in early cases should be to prevent tumour formation. In theory, keeping the animal out of the sunlight in the summer should afford a good measure of control but is rarely feasible. Reliable suncreams are helpful but application must be frequent to be effective. In practice, the most reliable treatment is amputation of the poorly protected ends of the pinnae. In more advanced cases where ulceration is marked and neoplasia suggested, total pinnectomy should be carried out. The tumours are locally invasive but metastasis is uncommon and the prognosis is good. Despite extensive surgery, the cosmetic appearance is normally satisfactory.

Temperature

Burns

Scalds over the dorsum running down the flanks and perilabial burns due to biting into electric wires are occasionally seen in cats. The treatment of these injuries follows that in any other domestic species.

Frost-bite

While frost-bite is rare in the UK, in extreme conditions the ears and, occasionally, the tail are susceptible to damage. The poorly insulated tips tend to be worst affected and are cool, pale and lack sensation but become reddened and painful as they thaw. In severe cases, the areas are sharply demarcated and may slough off.

Frozen tissue must be handled carefully and gently bathed with lukewarm water. Provided the tissue has not been completely devitalized, healing occurs quickly. Badly damaged areas should be removed surgically but this should not be carried out too early because more of the area may be potentially viable than at first may be imagined.

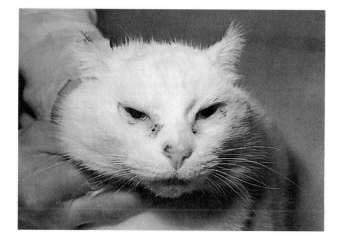

Fig. 10.8
Feline solar dermatitis. Eyelids and nasal skin in addition to the eartips are affected in this cat.

Diet

Nutritional factors which influence the skin are complex. As with any other system, good skin health requires a diet complete in all essential nutrients. Experimentally, skin lesions may be produced by feeding diets deficient in a number of factors but these rarely occur naturally. The most important results of incorrect nutrition are obesity and malnutrition.

Obesity

Obesity usually, but not always, results from overfeeding. Intertriginous dermatitis (axillae, groin, intermammary area) which may be accompanied by a secondary surface infection may result. The primary therapeutic aim is to reduce the cat's weight by dieting. Topical antibiotic/glucocorticoid creams may be palliative.

Malnutrition

malnutrition is occasionally encountered in neglected animals. The skin is usually dry, seborrhoeic, inelastic and may be more prone to secondary bacterial infections.

Fat-responsive dermatoses

This term is used in preference to fatty acid deficiency because affected animals are usually fed on balanced diets and have no evidence of maldigestion, malabsorption or liver disease. The true aetiology of the condition is unknown. Lesions consist of a dry or greasy coat with scaling and alopecia. Treatment consists of a fat supplement consisting of equal amounts (2.5–5 ml) of vegetable oil and animal fats (e.g. pork lard). Treatment may be required indefinitely.

Vitamin deficiency

Vitamin A deficiency is reported to cause poor coat, scaling and comedone formation.

Absolute or relative vitamin E deficiency may result in inflammation of the adipose tissue of the subcutis and elsewhere (pansteatitis, yellow fat disease) due to lack of its anti-oxidant properties. The condition may result from dietary lack of vitamin E or excessive dietary levels of unsaturated fatty acids. In addition to pain over the dorsum and abdomen, affected fat may feel firm and there may be pyrexia.

Diagnosis is suggested by physical examination, the presence of a raised white blood cell count (neutrophilia and eosinophilia) and is confirmed by biopsy. Treatment should include α-tocopherol supplements and dietary change. Glucocorticoids may be helpful to reduce inflammation.

INTERACTING FACTORS

ALLERGY

A number of agents may induce allergic responses in skin. However, contact allergy, with the exception of that caused by drugs and inhalant allergy, have not been confirmed in this species.

Parasites

Flea infestation is the commonest cause of allergic dermatitis in cats (Fig. 10.9). Immunological reactions have been suspected in tick-bite granulomata. Both of these states have been referred to previously.

Trombicula autumnalis infestation produces very variable reactions in different animals suggesting probable hypersensitivity.

Food allergy

Food allergy is rare in cats. Any item present in the diet is a potential allergen but reactions to sugars and minerals are very rare. The reactions are usually highly specific. The clinical appearance is very variable and although generalized pruritus is usually presnt, lesions may be localized (Fig. 10.10). Oedema may be seen and self-inflicted skin injury may result in exfoliation and skin damage. Occasionally, miliary dermatitis, eosinophilic plaques or pruritus without skin lesions may occur. Uncommonly, gastrointestinal symptoms resulting in colic, vomition or diarrhoea may be seen.

Some cases show a circulating eosinophilia but this is non-specific and diagnosis should be confirmed by test-meal investigation. Ideally, the diet should be formulated from foods not previously fed. With animals given a wide variety of foods, meat from a known pure source, e.g. beef, lamb or chicken, should be used together with rice. Commercial diets should not be used. Occasionally, short-term oral glucocortico-ids are necessary to reduce inflammation and pruritus prior to beginning the dietary testing. A favourable response should be seen in 2–3 weeks in correctly diagnosed cases. The specific allergen responsible is discovered by adding one constituent of the original diet for periods of 2 weeks until the symptoms occur. Skin testing for food allergens is of no value in the diagnosis of food allergy.

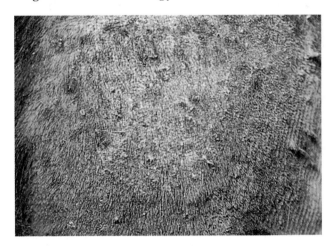

Fig. 10.9
Flea-bite hypersensitivity. The hair has been clipped from this cat's dorsal lumbo-sacral area to demonstrate the lesions.

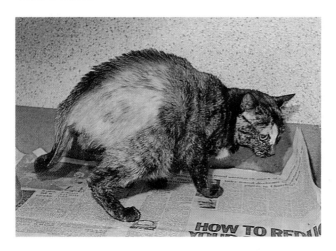

Fig. 10.10
Food allergy. Pruritus with resultant self inflicted injury caused hair fracture and alopecia over a large but solitary area.

Treatment relies ideally on avoidance of the offending allergen. Where owners are unwilling to comply with test-meal investigation or with its results, glucocorticoids must be relied on to produce some measure of control.

Drugs

Reports of drug eruptions in cats are few, probably because of the difficulties associated with confirming a diagnosis. On clinical grounds, allergic mechanisms are thought to be the most common cause of drug eruptions in man but the situation is not clear in animals. However, any drug may cause an eruption and there is no specific type of reaction for any one drug (Table 10.3).

In investigating such cases, all drugs should be stopped or changed to other unrelated compounds unless the risks of doing so outweigh the benefits to be obtained from diagnosis. Symptomatic therapy (glucocorticoids, antibiotics, etc.) mask diagnosis and should be avoided where possible.

Infection

The possibility that infectious agents, such as bacteria and fungi, may be allergenic as well as infectious in animals is

Table 10.3 Drug eruptions in the cat – incriminated drugs and resultant lesions.

Drug	Lesion
Sulfasoxizole	Miliary dermatitis, alopecia
Penicillin	Miliary dermatitis, urticaria – angioedema
Hetacillin	Multifocal alopecia, pruritus
Ampicillin	Multifocal alopecia, pruritus
	Toxic epidermal necrolysis
Tetracycline	Urticaria-angioedema
Cephaloridine	Toxic epidermal necrolysis
Neomycin	Contact dermatitis
Miconazole	Contact dermatitis
Dichlorvos	Contact dermatitis
Panleukopenia vaccine	Angioedema
Leukaemia virus antiserum	Toxic epidermal necrolysis

now being recognized and researched. Bacterial and fungal allergy has been suspected in cats but few details are available. Kerion formation is thought to be associated with fungal allergy.

Endoparasitism

Allergic dermatoses have been associated rarely with parasitism with roundworms, tapeworms and hookworms. Lesions are variable but pruritus is usually observed. Diagnosis is at present difficult. Faecal parasitological examination and response to treatment are suggestive but not conclusive evidence.

Diseases associated with auto-immunity

Recently, a number of skin diseases which are associated with auto-immunity have been described in the cat.

Pemphigus complex

The pemphigus complex is a group of chronic blistering diseases characterized clinically by involvement of skin and mucous membranes, histologically by acantholysis causing intraepidermal bullae and immunologically by the presence of circulating and tissue-bound auto-antibodies to intercellular epidermal antigens (Scott, 1980). A number of variants have been recognized in the cat – pemphigus vulgaris, pemphigus foliaceus and pemphigus erythematous – which are categorized, in the main, according to the level of acantholysis and immunofluorescence within the epidermis.

Cat epidermis is thin, bullae are therefore transient and erosions, ulcerations, epidermal collarettes together with erythema, crusting and scaling, are the usual presenting signs.

Diagnosis is based on histological examination of biopsies and direct immunofluorescence testing. Treatment with high-level glucocorticoids may induce remission but may require indefinite or intermittent use.

Systemic lupus erythematosus

Systemic lupus erythematous (SLE) is characterized by various types of autoantibody formation and variable involvement of a number of organ systems. While the aetiology is unknown, in man there are genetic predispositions. Reduction of suppressor T cell function and viral infection have been incriminated.

Very few cases of SLE have been recognized in the cat. Skin lesions described included erythema, vesicobullous eruptions, paronychia and pruritus. Diagnosis was made by positive antinuclear antibody tests, subcorneal blister formation in affected skin and the demonstration of immunoglobulin at the basement membrane of affected skin by direct immunofluorescence testing. Successful treatment and maintenance was with high level prednisolone.

Neoplasia

Skin tumours are relatively uncommon in cats (Table 10.4). They are frequently malignant and should be surgically removed early and routinely histologically examined. A more detailed list is set out in Table 10.5.

CONDITIONS OF UNKNOWN ORIGIN

EOSINOPHILIC GRANULOMA COMPLEX

The eosinophilic granuloma complex is a group of possibly related conditions affecting the skin and oral cavity. Scott (1975) has proposed a useful classification on clinical and histological critera:

(1) *Eosinophilic (rodent) ulcer* (Fig. 10.11) may occur on the skin and in the oral cavity but is usually found on the upper lip. The lesions are well demarcated, alopecic, reddish-brown or black with raised borders and an overlying, hardened crust and usually show no pruritus.

(2) *Eosinophilic plaque* (Fig. 10.2) may occur at any site but

Table 10.4 Frequency and distribution of feline skin tumours found in routine diagnosis over a 30-year period. (Courtesy of Department of Pathology, Royal (Dick) School of Veterinary Studies.)

Tumour	Number
Papilloma	5
Squamous cell carcinoma	9
Basal cell tumour	29
Sebaceous gland tumour	1
Sweat gland tumour	12
Ceruminous gland tumour	31
Melanoma	1
Fibrous tissue tumour	46
Vascular tumours	5
Mast cell tumours	20
Cutaneous lymphoreticular tumours	4
Epidermal cysts	6

Table 10.5 111Salient clinical features of feline skin tumours and tumour-like lesions.

Origin	Tumour	Age predisposition	Site(s) prevalence	Gross appearance	Behaviour	Treatment	Comments
EPITHELIAL	Papilloma	Middle-aged	None	Solitary, pedunculated, cauliflower-like	Benign, slow-growing may ulcerate and bleed	None or surgical excision	
	Squamous-cell carcinoma	Middle-aged to old	Unpigmented areas – external nares, eyelids, ears, lips	Solitary or multiple. Initially small erosion, firm consistency	Highly locally invasive. Late to metastasize	Radical surgical excision, including regional lymph nodes with radio-therapy where possible	Aetiology – ? ultra-violet light
	Basal cell	Middle-aged to old	Trunk, particularly neck and chest	Oval, well-circumscribed, often heavily pigmented	Benign slow growing. May ulcerate and bleed	None or surgical excision	
	Sebaceous gland	Middle-aged to old	None	Solitary, usually < 0.5 cm diameter, occasionally larger	Usually benign	Surgical excision	
	Sweat gland	Old	None	Solitary, usually 1–2 cm diameter, occasionally larger Fixed to overlying skin	Benign or malignant. Metastasize to regional lymph nodes and lungs	Early surgical excision	

continued

Table 10.5 *continued*

Origin	Tumour	Age predisposition	Site(s) prevalence	Gross appearance	Behaviour	Treatment	Comments
	Ceruminous gland	Middle-aged to old	Deep external auditory meatus	Frequently multiple, < 1 cm diameter, pinkish-grey, shiny, dome-shaped	All potentially malignant. Ulceration and secondary infection common	Surgical excision after lateral wall resection or vertical wall ablation	
	Melanoma	Old	None	Single, superficial, well-circumscribed, brown to black	Most metastasize to regional lymph nodes and lungs	Surgical excision +/- radiotherapy	
MESEN-CHYMAL	Fibrous tissue	Wide age range (< 4 months to 16 years)	~ 33% feet, ~ 33% nose, eyelids, ears ~ 33% scattered	*Fibroma* – well circumscribed, closely attached to overlying epidermis but mobile. Hair loss		Surgical excision	
				Fibrosarcoma – solitary (in cats < 4 months, multiple) poorly circumscribed, firm	Locally invasive May metastasize	Radical surgical excision. May recur locally	In some cases are caused by feline sarcoma virus
	Vascular	Adult to old	None	*Haemangioma* – solitary, small, (0.5–2 cm), oval, well circumscribed,	Do not metastasize	None or surgical excision	

			hair loss. May ulcerate and bleed		
			Malignant haemangioendothelioma – Rapidly growing, becoming large, friable and quickly ulcerate	Rapidly metastasize to lungs	Surgical excision difficult recur locally
Mast cell	Variable	None	Single or multiple, variably sized plaques, nodules or masses. May be pruritic if multiple. May ulcerate	Usually generalized with hepatomegaly and splenomegaly	Surgical excision for solitary tumours. Radiotherapy, chemotherapy (particularly glucocorticoids)
Lymphoreticular	Variable	None	Multiple cutaneous or subcutaneous nodules, plaques or ulcers. May be pruritic	Usually generalized with lymphomegaly. Fatal	None
Epidermal (non-neoplastic) Epidermal cyst	None	Neck and trunk	Usually solitary, occasionally multiple, well-circumscribed, rounded, fluctuating to firm, filled with white to grey, caseous material. Some are intensely pigmented	Benign	Surgical excision

is commonly seen over the ventral abdomen, thorax and medial thighs. Lesions are well demarcated, raised, alopecic, moist, bright red, eroded or ulcerated areas. Pruritus is usually marked.

(3) *Linear granuloma* occurs at any site but is commonly found over the posterior hindlimbs and within the oral cavity. Lesions are well demarcated, raised, firm, yellow or yellowish-pink, linear or nodular. They are frequently asymptomatic but oral forms may cause drooling of saliva and dysphagia.

The aetiology of the eosinophilic granuloma complex is

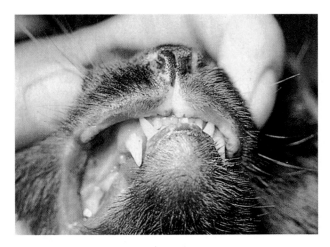

Fig. 10.11
Eosinophilic granuloma complex: eosinophilic ulcer. Surgical excision was curative.

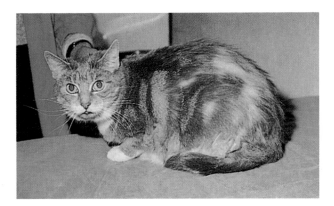

Fig. 10.12
Eosinophilic granuloma complex: eosinophilic plaque. Remission was induced and maintained with prednisolone.

unknown and may be mutlifactorial, possibly as a result of pruritus in some cases. The author has diagnosed flea-bite hypersensitivity and food allergy which were presented as eosinophilic plaques. Genetic influences have also been suggested. Causal bacteria, fungi or viruses have not been isolated although, as previously noted, Neufield *et al.* (1980) identified as a picornavirus in affected tissues. Some form of "immunological mediation" has been suggested but explanatory details were notably lacking.

A circulatory eosinophilia is usually seen in the plaque form but much less commonly in other forms of the condition. A non-specific (30–40%) increase in gammaglobulins may occur but definitive diagnosis rests on histological examination of affected tissues. Tissue eosinophilia is seen in the plaque and oral linear granuloma types but less commonly in other forms.

Prior to terming the disease idiopathic and resorting to purely symptomatic therapy, possible precipitating causes (flea infestation, food allergy, etc.) should be investigated and treated accordingly. Oral, systemic or intralesional glucocorticoids or oral progestogens such as megoestrol acetate, are effective in most cases, but it is impossible to predict which will be the most suitable for any individual. Intermittent high dose or long-term low dose therapy may be required. Early surgical excision is recommended for medically resistant lip ulcer. This treatment is quick, effective and surprisingly rarely troubled by wound breakdown. Other possible lines of therapy include cryosurgery, radiotherapy and immunopotentiating agents (e.g. levamisole or thiabendazole). Spontaneous regression of lesions has been noted.

ACNE

Feline acne (Fig. 10.13) is a poorly understood condition with no breed, sex or age predisposition. Genetic predisposition, failure to clean or incorrect eating habits seem unlikely causes and it is probably linked with abnormal sebaceous gland function, where their density is high.

Patients are presented with comedone formation over the chin extending perilabially, sometimes as far as the lip commissures. In most cases, there is no pruritus or pain but rarely there may be secondary infection with pustule formation, oedema and furunculosis.

In many cases, no therapy is required but comedones may be extracted manually or with commercial human "blackhead" extractors. Ethyl alcohol (50–100%) as a defatting agent, proprietary human astringents or keratolytics, such as sulphur or selenium sulphide, may be helpful. Maintenance therapy is usually required. In infected cases, the affected area should be clipped, the comedones evacuated and systemic antibiotics given.

STUD TAIL

The supra-caudal organ of the cat is an area of unique skin situated dorsally on the tail, consisting of modified sebaceous glands. "Stud tail" is characterized by overproduction of sebum by these glands resulting in a yellowish-grey accumulation of oily material, matting of hair and variable degrees of alopecia. The condition is one of purebred cats and purebred crosses, mainly in entire males but it also occurs in females and neuters. The aetiology is unknown but has been suggested to be due to confinement with resultant failure to groom.

Treatment, if required, is similar to that for non-infected acne but may have to be given indefinitely. The effects of a greater degree of freedom should be evaluated.

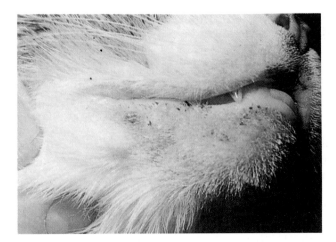

Fig. 10.13
Feline acne. Area has been clipped to demonstrate the lesions.

LIP OEDEMA

Lip oedema is uncommon and of unknown aetiology. It affects the lower lip and occasionally the chin, usually independently of acne. The affected skin is swollen, firm, smooth and shiny without pruritus or pain.

Treatment is usually not required and, in fact, has little effect. Spontaneous (although frequently slow) resolution is the rule.

MILIARY DERMATITIS

While this condition is certainly multifactorial, its aetiology is needlessly controversial, being in most cases due to flea-bite hypersensitivity and responding to comprehensive flea control measures in the absence of other treatments. Such cases also respond well to megoestrol acetate without attempts at flea control, explaining, in part, the commonly held, erroneous belief that the condition is of endocrine origin. The mode of action of the drug in such cases is unknown and, while it may occasionally have a place in aiding resolution of severe cases, it should never be used as a substitute for parasiticidal therapy which should always be the first line of approach.

Other possible causes include *Cheyletiella* infestation, pediculosis, dermatomycosis, food allergy and drug eruption. Very occasional cases are idiopathic and these can be difficult to control with either glucocorticoids or progestogens.

PLASMA CELL PODODERMATITIS

A condition of unknown aetiology, plasma cell pododermatitis, is characterized by enlargement and softening of the metacarpal, metatarsal and, less commonly, the digital pads of one or more feet. The lesions may ulcerate but pruritus, pain and lameness are usually absent.

Diagnosis is based on physical signs and histopathological examination of biopsies which reveals plasma cell and neutrophil infiltration of the dermis and underlying adipose tissue. Non-specific abnormalities are variable but include leucocytosis, lymphocytosis, neutrophilia with left shift and raised globulin levels. On post-mortem examination, there may be plasma cell infiltration of viscera and amyloidosis of kidneys and liver.

The condition may resolve spontaneously. Response to glucocorticoids, antibiotics and bandaging is variable.

TOXIC EPIDERMAL NECROLYSIS

Toxic epidermal necrolysis (Lyell syndrome) is a recently recognized condition characterized by systemic signs, such as depression, anorexia, pyrexia and skin lesions. These consist of painful mucocutaneous bullae and ulcers, epidermal collarettes and a positive Nikolsky sign (apparently normal skin that wrinkles on rubbing). In man, it may be associated with drug eruption, systemic disease or be idiopathic. In the cat, cases have been recognized during treatment with ampicillin, cephaloridine and leukaemia virus antiserum.

Diagnosis is confirmed by biopsy. Treatment includes high dosage of glucocorticoids, general support and correction of the underlying cause.

ACKNOWLEDGEMENTS

The author acknowledges the helpful comments of Professor J. T. Baxter during the preparation of this paper. He is grateful to Mr K. W. Head for the information on frequency and distribution of tumours and his consecutive criticism. Mr R. K. Thomson produced the photographs.

REFERENCES AND FURTHER READING

Dawson, C. O. & Noddle, B. M. (1968). *Journal of Small Animal Practice* **9**, 613.

Muller G. H. & Kirk, R. W. (1976). *Small Animal Dermatology*, 2nd edn. W. B. Saunders, Philadelphia.

Neufield, J. L., Burton, L. & Jeffrey, K. R. (1980). *Veterinary Pathology* **17**, 97.

Scott, D. W. (1975). *Journal of the American Animal Hospitals Association* **11**, 261.

Scott, D. W. (1980). *Journal of the American Animal Hospitals Association* **16**, 333.
Thoday, K. L. (1979). *In Practice* **1**, 5.
Thoday, K. L. (1980). *British Veterinary Journal* **137**, 133.
Thomsett, L. R., Baxby, D. & Denham, E. M. H. (1978). *Veterinary Record* **103**, 567.
Wright, A. I. (1973) *The Veterinary Annual* (eds C. S. G. Grunsell & F. W. G. Hill) 15th edn. J. Wright, Bristol.

Index